Cover Art
By Fay Risner

ISBN 1438244991
EAN 13 - 9781438244990

Books By Fay Bookstore Website
http://www.booksbyfaystore.weebly.com

1

Reader Reviews

I enjoyed your book. It was very touching. Thanks for sharing.

Diana Roy
Keystone, Iowa

I certainly am blessed to be a recipient of your book. The book is a great resourceful collection of ideas and suggestions.

Jurine Moore
Marion, Iowa

The woman, who I mentioned in my previous correspondence has used excerpts from your book for inservices. I plan on doing the same with credit to you in my lecture material on Alzheimer's.

Rosemarie Van WilligeRN
Montezuma, Iowa

I hope you get recognized for your wonderful writing.

Kristi Struve R.N.
Mt. Auburn, Iowa

I read, I learned, I laughed and I cried.

Judy Hupfeld
Coralville, Iowa

Acknowledgment

This book is dedicated to my parents for teaching me by example how to make lemonade out of life's lemons.

Also to Sue Meyer, a friend, who showed me an example of a genuinely caring caregiver.

Contents

Open A

Window

An Alzheimer's Caregiver's

Handbook

Fay Risner

Preface

From our earliest memories we start to care about the well being of those that are closest to us. As adults we are destine to become caregivers to someone; first to our children, then elderly parents, a spouse, other relatives, in-laws or friends that need our help. Before we know it our days are consumed with bathing, grooming, dressing, feeding, toileting, dispensing medication, watching over and entertaining a care receiver for twenty four/seven.

Each day, we rush through the caregiving tasks at hand while thinking ahead to the endless tasks yet to be done. With a sinking feeling, we realize that there just isn't enough time in the day. We just don't have enough stamina to complete everything. Our mind might be willing, but our body isn't. Our busy and practical caregiving role leaves little time to open windows to create and savor the moments that make caregiving rewarding, or moments that we need to work on to make life more worthwhile for the people who need our care. We are so focused on their physical needs and busy mourning the loss of their familiar, former self that we forget to savor what is left of the special person that we care for. We should cherish the person that is now while there is still time.

Besides the stories in my book that show ways to help someone with Alzheimer's disease, I have included some introspective essays that share with the reader my feelings about caring for people. All in one way or another designed to put *care* back in caregiving.

In this book are moments I call opening a window. I might not have noticed that I opened those windows when caring for residents in a nursing home if it hadn't been for the experience of taking care of my father. Being a caregiver on a personal level gave me an insight I wouldn't have had otherwise. Caring for Dad helped me realize as a professional caregiver I was consumed with taking care of the physical needs for the residents, but people with Alzheimer's disease need more than that. They need caregivers to care enough to inspire and exercise their brains so even if it's for a brief moment, we've help to let their thoughts, trapped in the shell that has become them, escape to shine out of the windows in their brain.

With five million people in this country suffering from Alzheimer's disease and millions more needing our help in the years to come, we need to be prepared, but we aren't. When the younger generations come on board as caregivers at nursing homes, they have so much to learn about taking care of people with Alzheimer's disease. Training is very important whether it be watching an experienced caregiver or reading anything that you can get your hands on that will help you succeed in making a better day for someone with Alzheimer's.

Up until now we have been using the tried and failed methods to get to the successful approaches. All the while, our efforts to learn are at the expense of confused and frustrated people who become uncontrollable and on medication, because they can't express themselves any other way. All they want is caregivers who understand what is happening to their brain and know how to help them when they can't express themselves or help themselves. People with Alzheimer's are depending on us, the caregivers. It's time for all of us to figure out what works to create the best quality of life we can for the people with Alzheimer's.

There is plenty of documentation for what works and what doesn't to educate every caregiver. Find it, read and practice what you read. Make life as problem free as you can for someone with Alzheimer's. Even if they can't tell you how much they appreciate your thoughtfulness and help. I know they feel it deep inside themselves.

This book is designed to help caregivers understand what Alzheimer's disease does to people. I hope to give you some idea about how to help people with this dreadful disease.

The list is as follows

To use for training sessions for caregivers taking care of residents in long term care or on an individual basis in Home Health Care.

For family members who need educated about Alzheimer's so they understand why a person acts they way they do. Once they understand, they will be better caregivers.

For use at Alzheimer's support groups to help educate caregivers.

1.

The Key Is Understanding

Because I chose to be a certified nurse aide (CNA) that makes her living in a care center, I've always thought of myself as a caring person. I believed I was good at my job. It took helping my mother care for my father, who had Alzheimer's disease, to make me realize that I had much more to learn. After my father's death, I returned to work at the care center and began to see the residents in a new way. I felt the need to dig deeper into my grab bag full of skills and emotions I carried inside me to put the emphasis on *care* in caregiving.

Times have changed. We care for and treat the physical ailments of frail, elderly people as we always have, but now we're caring for people with Alzheimer's disease and other related dementia. With the increase of this disease, we have had to learn new skills and terminology. It takes practice to perfect skills CNAs learn for the most part through on the job experience. Just when we think we have it down pat, the procedure that worked once on a person won't work anymore, because of the changes in that person's brain.

Since Alzheimer's disease affects each person differently as the disease damages the brain the procedure the caregiver practiced on someone else might not work at all on the next person.

We need to be fast thinking and flexible enough to switch to another approach. Above all, we need to be patient, calm, soft spoken and act like we really care. A variety of tried examples that have worked for other caregivers doesn't hurt either. That's why it's important for the caregiver at home or in long term care to research all the approaches to find the reason why something works for someone with Alzheimer's disease.

An important part of taking care of someone is knowing that person's likes, dislikes, hobbies and life stories. A relative taking care of that person has it made in that regard. Long term caregivers have to play a guessing game which may lead the person to frustration, anger, and a bad day. Find out from relatives what you need to know to keep the person from going home or trying to find their children. Help that person enjoy a conversation about a subject she like. Memories may have faded, but you bring up something that was a pleasant memory for her. See how fast she begins to take interest and add her thoughts to the conversation.

Contact your local Alzheimer's office and ask for educational materials, books and videos from their lending library that are loaned out free for a month and get the free pamphlets to give family and friends to educate them. The Association mails the material to caregivers that aren't able to come to the office.

Caregivers feel the need to be clinical as we rush to make it through each day whether it be at home or working an eight hour shift in a facility. There's no time to spare when we have a schedule to keep. Let something slow us down and it has a snowball effect to screw up our schedule for the rest of the day. So we watch the clock, try to keep on schedule, and at the same time do a good job of caring for the loved one at home, or the residents in a nursing home. That rush - rush attitude only creates a frustrating atmosphere for the person with AD. Their brain doesn't process fast anymore. They need much more time to digest what is going on around them or what is said to them. They need time to think about their response to us. We need to slow down for the person with AD.

That fast moving caregiver was me until I helped Mom take care of my father in his home. Now I see images of Dad as he was through the long, ten years he suffered with Alzheimer's from an open window in my healthy brain's memory room. Comparing my experience with my father to the people I have cared for since has changed how I view my job. Five million people have Alzheimer's disease. In the next few years that number will triple as the baby boomers become retirement age. That means health care workers may very soon have the experience of caring for someone in their family who has Alzheimer's disease as well as being flooded with a rising number of residents with dementia in long term care. We need to get our caregiving techniques down pat. Time for that is running out.

However, caregivers don't have to have someone close to them afflicted with Alzheimer's disease for them to develop an empathy for people who have the disease. As professional caregivers, take the time to get to know the people you're caring for. Think about the dreadful, terminal road ahead of them. As the saying goes, "Walk a mile in their shoes. See how it feels".

The key to caring is getting to know and understand what a person with Alzheimer's is all about. Not just what you see on the surface, but the person behind the curtain of Alzheimer's disease. -- Fay Risner

2.

Windows In The Brain

This is my description of what happens to a person's brain when they have Alzheimer's disease.

When we are born, our brain is full of well lit, airy, vacant rooms with an open window in each one. Knowledge and experiences flow through the open windows to fill the rooms as we grow, and flow back out as we mentally call on them to create the type of human being we become. Imagine if by the time you are in your sixties, you was to find yourself searching for a thought in the memory room. You find that the room had become dark, the drapes are drawn. You strain to see the familiar object you are searching for in your mind, trying to remember what it looked like the last time you saw it, but you can't find that object in the dark.

That's what happens to a person who is afflicted with Alzheimer's disease. One such person was a large framed, boisterous farmer who spoke with a loud voiced, salty vocabulary. First, the memory room in his brain became dark, then other rooms darkened as they were covered with a black shroud called plaque that continued slowly to spread from room to room.

As it entered the open windows, the plaque closed them, and the drapes drew shut to put out the light. As this happened to the farmer, he became a shell of the man his family and friends once knew and was admitted to a care center. In time, he forgot how to feed himself, had trouble swallowing, couldn't do his activities of daily living skills, and could barely stand long enough to transfer from the bed to the wheelchair. The only vocabulary he had left was loud, frustrated profanity unless he chose to parrot short sentences he heard from the aides such as "It's time to eat.", or "It's bedtime.".

There came a time when the farmer quit repeating what he heard. His face became expressionless, and his eyes stared vacantly. I was sure that most of the windows in his brain had shut, became locked, and would never reopen again. I was wrong!

Since the farmer was in his room most of the day, I had taken to sitting him in the living room with the other residents after the evening meal. I hoped people talking, and Vanna White flashing across the television screen would stimulate his mind. As time went by, I gave up hope that what I was doing would trigger anything in the farmer that I would see outwardly, but I consoled myself with the idea that I didn't know what was happening inside those dark rooms in his brain. You know how the window frames in an old house doesn't fit quite tight, and a small amount of air seeps between the sills and the frames? I thought maybe that might be how the windows in the farmer's mind were working so I felt I shouldn't give up trying to stimulate him even if I couldn't see I was helping him.

One evening at bedtime, I pushed the farmer's wheelchair across the living room. As we neared a visitor, sitting by his wife, the visitor reached out his hand and patted the farmer's knee.

"Hello," the visitor greeted.

"Hello," the farmer returned in his booming voice, and he called the man by name. The blank expression on the farmer's face changed to one of joy at seeing an old friend.

"He knows you!" I exclaimed in surprise as I realized the farmer recognized the visitor, and he actually spoke

5

without repeating another person's sentence. The farmer's eyes remained focused on the visitor.

"He should," the visitor replied. "We've been friends for years, and we were both on the board of a business in town for a long time, weren't we?"

"Yes," the farmer answered with gusto.

I could see a calm look of contentment on his face as the memory room's window crept open to let out the memories I had been so sure were trapped forever in darkness.

"We went to a lot of those board meetings together," the visitor continued. He patted the farmer's knee again as he said, "This is the man who made a lot of the important decision at the meetings, didn't you?"

Tears welled up in the farmer's eyes as he struggled to grasp memories long forgotten. I hated to see him so sad, and I didn't want this to be an uncomfortable situation for him or the visitor so I tried to add a little humor to the conversation.

"Oh, sure! Were those important decisions what time to go get the beer after the meetings were over?"

Both men laughed at my teasing as the farmer slowly boomed out, "Yes!"

Then I explained to the visitor that it was the farmer's bedtime so he had to leave. By the time I had wheeled the farmer the short distance down the hall into his room and closed the door, hiss face was expressionless again. His eyes stared vacantly, focused on the drapes behind his bed which were closed across the window just like the pair that darkened the window that had shut again in his mind.

For all my trying, I hadn't been the one to open a window for the farmer, but that's all right because I was there to see it happen, and that was enough incentive to make me keep trying.

One inspiring source to read for caregivers is Jolene Brackey's book titled Creating Moments Of Joy. Her website is another place to check out for helpful information which is http://www.enhancedmoments.com. She always has helpful articles designed to make pleasant days for people with Alzheimer's. I was thrilled when Jolene used my Open A Window story in the third edition of her Creating Moments Of Joy. She even autographed her book for me. That for me was a moment of joy I hope I never forget.

When one door closes, another opens -- Alexander Graham Bell

3.

Opening A Window

We never know what will open a window in the brain, but that doesn't mean we should quit trying. How would you like to be shut in a dark room where the only way out is a locked window that you can't figure out how to open? That's the way it is for a person whose brain is being destroyed by Alzheimer's disease.

It's up to us as caregivers to look for ways to open those locked windows in the brain. If by chance you, as a caregiver, figure out what "motion detector" will trigger the opening of a window, don't expect it to work again. You may have to come up with a different "motion detector" next time because of the changes in that person's brain.

However be prepared for the moment the window does open, because it will only be for a brief time. Wham! The window closes again. Please don't be too busy being a caregiver to miss the moment when it happens like the moment I remember in this story.

When my newborn animals hit the ground each spring,

I box up a lamb and a goat -- literally put my babies in a cardboard box, tie it shut with baling twine, then transport them in the trunk of my car into the care center. I used to set the box in the front passenger seat. With the air on, I thought I was doing the babies a favor. One day, I didn't tie the box top tight enough. On the way into the nursing home, the lamb and goat decided to stand up. They bumped the box top with their heads, and the flaps slipped out from under the baling twine. The minute, those two saw daylight, they were out of that box and in the floor beside me. I'll let you imagine the rest of the story. It has something to do with giving the inside of my car a good scrubbing when I got home.

Once I get to the nursing home, I place the box (with high sides) in a wheelchair or on a moving cart. I unwrap the babies for the residents to pet and watch their expressions while I listen to their stories of long ago farming days. Maybe the person lived in town and wasn't too impressed with my animals. That's the person that appreciated my woos about my car needing a good scrubbing and airing when I got back home. Either way, the time I spent sharing something in my life that gave me pleasure gave them a few moments of pleasures ten fold.

That's why what happened to Ellen that day, I wish some of the other caregivers I worked with could have witnessed.

Always unresponsive and staring at the wall, Ellen, in the late stage of Alzheimer's, sat with her limp hands in her lap while I positioned the baby animals as close as I could get them to her.

"Look what I brought for you to see, Ellen."

No response.

"Can you look down at my box, Ellen?"

No response.

As long as the wheelchair was in motion the babies stayed content, but the moment I stopped, they grew restless, trying to jump out of the box. The lamb reared up, stuck his front hooves on the kid's back, knocking the goat to his knees. The kid let out a loud, screaming protest, "Baa a a!".

Only then did Ellen looked down to see where the strange noise came from. Her eyes widened and lit up as she focused on the animals. Smiling, she asked, "What have you got there?"

"I brought my baby animals for you to see. Want to pet them?"

I picked up Ellen's limp hand and laid it on the lamb's soft, woolly topknot. I watched as her fingers cupped around the lamb's head while she smiled at him. The kid's cry and touching the lamb's head were triggers for Ellen, bringing her awake to what was happening at the moment. ELLEN was very well aware of what she was doing. She enjoyed that moment.

I realized that I'd opened a window for Ellen, but also, I knew it would shut again as soon as I left the room. That's the power Alzheimer's disease had over her mind. No matter how hard she tried to stay focused on what was going on around her without a trigger to jog her memory, her mind was empty.

Most but not all of the residents in our nursing home have a rural background. It may have been they were farmers or they grew up on a farm. Perhaps, they had enjoyable visits at their grandparents farms. That's why they react to my baby animals. Almost always, a resident who had a urban background, if they like animals, will enjoy the farm animals, too. But once in awhile that if is a very big IF. Some people just don't care about being around animals. They might notice the barn odor and want to stay away from the smell. Then there are the residents that think my babies are dogs. One man pointed to my black lamb and told me he once had a dog just like that one. My response was, "That must have been a very nice dog." As long as the man enjoyed watching my animals that was the important thing, not that he had forgotten what a dog looked like.

What lies behind us and what lies before us are tiny matters compared to what lies within us. -- *Ralph Waldo Emerson*

4.

I Have Alzheimer's

There must not be anything much worse in this world than being afraid all the time of doing or saying something wrong because of confusion or feeling lost. People with Alzheimer's feel as if they can't do or say the simplest things the right way. They know that fact because everyone corrects them. Have you ever wondered what was going on in a person with Alzheimer's mind? Come along with me. Let's pretend to open a window in one woman's mind who lives in a care center and peek in.

I motioned to the two people in white to come to me, because I wanted to talk to them.

One stopped just long enough to ask me if I had a problem.

I said, "Yes."

She asked, "Are you still hungry?"

Not being sure what the word was that I should use to let the aide know I wanted food, I took a guess. "No."

I wondered where she got that *still* hungry business. I

can't remember when I last ate. Of course, I'm hungry. I don't know why that woman bothered to ask. She hurried away and never did bring me anything to eat.

The people dressed in white showed up fast enough when I got hot and unbuttoned my blouse while I was watching television in the living room. One of them buttoned my blouse back up. She told me if I tried one more trick like that, I'd have to go to my room. I have news for them! This is my room. I just wish all these strangers sitting around me in my living room would go home. I need peace and time to be alone. This place is too noisy with all these other people here.

Sitting in the same hard chair for so long was tiresome. I decided to stretch my legs. From the window I could see it was a pretty day. I wanted to go outside for a walk. I opened the door. What I thought was the fire alarm blared around me. When I heard that loud noise, it scared me. I tried to escape out the door fast, but people in white rushed at me from every direction. Two of them walked me back to my chair, and one of them told me in a not too friendly tone to stay put.

I couldn't do that, because by then I had to find the bathroom. I started to look for one, but this house of mine is a big place with lots of rooms. Somehow I have forgotten how to find my way around. The first door I opened, I smelled food. The good smells made my stomach growl, reminding me I was hungry, but a strange woman told me to go away. I went in several other rooms looking for the bathroom but found only beds there. Some with people sleeping in them. One woman screamed at me to get out.

Two people in white grabbed me, escorting me faster than I like to walk back to that same old, uncomfortable chair. They sat me down, and one of them said in a harsh voice, "Now stay here this time!"

I wet my pants. I've not done that since I was a baby. I feel so embarrassed and ashamed of myself. Finally now that it was too late, two of those people in white showed up to take me to the bathroom to change my clothes. One of them told me in a patronizing tone that it was all right. It wasn't my fault that I wet my pants. I have Alzheimer's disease. In my mind, there isn't an excuse for being incontinent.

I feel so frustrated, because I don't understand what's happening to me. It makes me wonder if these people in white have the same disease they tell me I have, because if they were to ask me, I'd say there is defiantly something wrong with all of them.

We have to work on communication with a person who has dementia. It's not just what the person says, but what they can't say. Sometimes body language clues us in on what they need or want.

Perhaps just getting to know someone with Alzheimer's disease can help us decipher that particular individual's needs if we aren't too busy to pay attention. One resident that I took care of was a very dear friend. I knew her extremely well. When her language sounded foreign (word salad) with only an English word sprinkle in the sentences, I watched her face. I picked up on the words I recognized. Sure sometimes it was guess work, but most of the time, I was able to carry a conversation with my friend that kept her thinking that she had communicated successfully. I could tell she was thinking in English but just couldn't speak in English. How frustrating is that when the person you want to talk to looks at you with no understanding about what you're trying to convey? I knew frustrated and alone was how my friend felt when one day she said very clearly to me, "I always like it when you help me. We can talk. No one else will talk to me."

If you can't pick up enough to know what the resident tried to say, why not carrying the conversation. Try talking about the nice day or compliment the person on what they are wearing and how nice their hair is fixed. Do your homework so you know what the person takes pleasure in hearing. You make the conversation so maybe that resident doesn't have to struggle to make one with you.

The key is stop treating the residents differently. They

aren't just the resident in room 321 in bed 1 that needs us to do all their ADLs (Activity Of Daily Living Skills). They realize more than we give them credit for. The struggle for them is to convey their thoughts. Listen. Give them time to speak no matter how slowly the words come out. They need to know you hear them and value their opinions.

5.

The Lady Who Cried

An aide walked by Emma's room. She noticed that Emma was sitting in her recliner, crying again.

"Look. Emma is on another crying jag," the aide said nonchalantly to her coworker.

"Leave her alone for a while. She'll be okay. It's Alzheimer's disease that causes her to cry," said the other aide with the know it all wisdom of someone who had seen this lady cry often.

These two aides didn't know Emma in her past life before she entered the care center. She was a happy-go-lucky widow that enjoyed life and had a good time no matter where she was.

As she grew older, her large house became too much for her to take care of so she sold it and down sized her possessions to fit into an assisted living apartment. Emma needed to adjust to living in a smaller home, but that wasn't to be. Often she would go into other people's apartments when she was looking for her own. Confusion about where she was and what was going on around her became a big part of her life.

The doctor diagnosed Emma with Alzheimer's disease. She had to give up most of her possessions and her freedom when she moved into one room in a care center. The room was just big enough to hold the only familiar possessions she had left: a recliner, an end table and a radio.

If those aides had realized how much better her life used to be, understood how unhappy Emma was to have to move to the care center, and if they had thought about how much worse the situation was going to get as Alzheimer's disease progressed, that would have made their eyes tear up right along with Emma.

Once when I went in to comfort Emma while she was crying, I thought I could do so by talking to her about a happy subject so I said, "One of your daughters came to visit yesterday. Was that Donna or Emily?"

Emma said sadly, "I don't know for sure."

"That's all right. It doesn't matter," I said, patting her hand.

"Well, it does to me. I don't know why I can't remember," she wailed and began to cry again.

"It's okay. We love you the way you are," I comforted.

Always a loving mother even with Alzheimer's, Emma put her hands to her cheeks and said, "But it does matter to my kids."

No words seemed to work. It was my hug that gave her comfort.

Several months later as Alzheimer's disease destroyed more of her brain, I asked Emma why she was crying. She said, "I don't know. I just feel like crying."

Even though she didn't know why she cried, Emma carried a sad feeling around with her all the time, ready at any moment to burst to the surface. We labeled her crying as a symptom of Alzheimer's disease. Sure Emma had AD so she had gotten to the point that she couldn't remember what made her sad, but don't you agree with her? Whether she could remember or not, she had a reason to cry.

Her caregivers needed to do whatever it took to make her feel better like listen to her fears, or try to get her onto a happier subject, or give her a hug to let her know she is not alone. Let her know you care. If nothing else worked, it's all right to leave her alone for a while to cry until she vented her pent up emotions. The main thing is instead of excusing Emma's sadness as Alzheimer's as they walked by her room, the aides should have taken the time to care.

As her caregivers, they should have given some thought to how hard it was for Emma to make it through each day when confusion, sad thoughts, worries and fears hung over her head like a dark, storm cloud ready to release more teardrops.

I was present one night when Emma helped console another resident that had the same type of problems that she had. Emma and three other women were at the dining room table for the evening meal. As I listened to their conversation, I could see Emma was all too aware of her own memory limitations at that moment.

One of the ladies, a former school teacher, pronounced every word correctly with an air of someone highly educated, asked for a cup of coffee. I poured it for her. She drank about half of the cup, and continued to eat her meal. Later she motioned for me to come to her. In a displeased voice, she said slowly, "I asked for a cup of coffee some time ago, and I didn't get it."

"Yes, I poured your coffee," I said, holding her cup over so she could see it was still half full.

"I'm so sorry," she apologized to me. "I don't know what's the matter with me. I forgot that you brought me the coffee."

"It's all right," Emma sympathized, patting the lady's hand. "We get confused sometimes."

See how easy it was for Emma to put herself in that

woman's shoes. She knew exactly how the woman felt. At that moment as Emma watched the other woman, she realized that forgetting happened often to each of them. With a certain dread, she had to feel that the next time it would be her turn to be confused.

Keep in mind, telling someone that you did pour the coffee might not be enough to make them believe you. They are always right. Remember that. Apologize for forgetting to pour her coffee and fill the cup up. She is happy, and you didn't remind her she has a problem with her memory which made her feel bad or worried.

I read this joke in a newspaper column, and it stuck with me. Keep in mind, it's all right to laugh even though we feel for the people who struggle with confusion. The joke was meant to be funny, but it reminds me just how confused a person's mind can become.

Two aides were walking with a male resident in the nursing home yard. A flock of birds flew over them, and one dropped a deposit on the man's bald head.

One of the aides said, "Stay right here. I'll go get some toilet paper."

As she rushed away, the elderly man turned to the other aide and said, "She's kind of dingy, isn't she? That bird will be long gone before she gets back with the paper."

Prediction is very difficult, especially about the future -- Niels Bohr

6.

The Imaginary Trip

Henry, a quiet, polite, gentle man, and his wife, Ruth, moved into the care center. Ruth had Alzheimer's. Henry had been her caregiver for years. It wasn't long after the couple came that we noticed Henry's confusion, possibly from years of stressful caregiving. Then Ruth passed away. It was hard for Henry to adjust to not having his wife (his friend and soul mate) near him after taking care of her for years. The constant sad reminder of his loss was the empty bed across the room from his.

One night I was helping Henry do his evening ADLs (activity of daily living skills) in the bathroom. I noticed he seemed to be in a more jovial mood than he had been lately. As we walked across the room toward his bed, Henry exclaimed, "This is a wonderful place to stay. You people are so accommodating and take such good care of me. I really appreciate what you do for me."

I felt like he had given me a big imaginary pat on the back. "Well, thank you for saying so. I'm glad you like it here. We like having you stay with us."

Henry stopped and gave his bed an amazed stare. "This looks just like the bed I've been sleeping in at the other place I've been at. It's such a nice bed."

"This is the bed you sleep in," I slowly exclaimed, wondering what Henry was getting at.

"Now I know you are all wonderful here. You had my bed shipped all the way to Los Angeles!"

"We're in California?" I asked, surprised by his answer.

"Yes, this is a hotel in Los Angeles," Henry informed me.

"Why did we come to Los Angeles?" Now I was curious to find out the rest of his story.

"My nephew has been wanting me to come visit him so he sent me a plane ticket, and got me reservations in this hotel. Now you people have shipped my comfortable bed to me. This is great!"

It began to register with me that Henry didn't think I was his traveling companion but a hotel maid. That's not exactly the way I'd want to spend my time on a trip with him to California, but this was Henry's imaginary trip not mine.

I helped him into bed, covered him up and turned off the lights. I had played along, saying all the right things when I entered Henry's reality. If I had tried to tell him the truth, he'd have been upset, because he wouldn't have believed me. He may have refused to go to bed, or maybe he wouldn't have been able to go to sleep. He'd have started to grieve all over again when he remembered why the bed across the room was empty.

In the morning, I knew Henry would wake up to the way things were again as he knew them, but I'd helped Henry get a peaceful night's sleep for one night. He'd ignored the empty bed across the room, because he thought it was in a hotel. In the morning, the memory of that pleasant trip would be erased from his mind. The empty bed might again remind him of his loss, but for a few peaceful moments he had in a troubling time, Henry needed me to go along with him on his imaginary trip.

Not long after that evening, Henry was moved to another room where there were no reminders of his painful loss. That doesn't mean that he didn't grieve the loss of his wife once in a while, but the constant reminder of an empty bed across from him was gone.

What I did was enter his reality. I was in the world he was in at the moment. When a person regresses to a safer place in his life away from today, we need to go along with that person. For them, the place in their mind is a comfortable place with happier memories. We need to join them in their safe place. Doing this is a little like acting in a play. Once the caregiver gets the hang of it being in the person with Alzheimer's play can be fun. Just settle into the person's place, go along with his thinking and enjoy the tour of his world as he lived it years before when he was a young and healthy person.

Usually with the regression, their memories are only happy moments. All the trivial happenings in their life has been forgotten if there wasn't an emotion attached to them. In their confusion, the safe place to be is with the pleasant memories of a loving spouse, small children, and a secure home.

Not all the memories they recall are safe and happy. With one woman I recall, the emotion that kept haunting her from the past was not happiness but worry. She continually wanted to be reassured that she had a room at the nursing home. Over and over, she wanted to hear that she still had long term life insurance to cover her care. On the surface, her repetition of the same questions was a symptom of Alzheimer's disease that I was use to hearing.

When a member of her family asked me why the woman asked the same questions over after they had been answered, I gave this explanation. Her brain is like a loaded computer that can take in no more information. The computer in her mind had filled up several years before. Because this woman had struggled to make ends meet for so long, worries were on her mind always. She couldn't reason that she was safe and shouldn't worry about a roof over her head or her finances so she asked the questions to anyone she saw. But since she couldn't retain the answers, she kept asking the same questions over and over.

What I felt was behind her questions was as she regressed back to younger days, this woman didn't feel the happy emotion that would bring back the pleasant memories in her present life. She regressed into a place where she was a young widow with two small children. In her past, she worked hard and worried about keeping a roof over her family's head and paying the bills.

Trying to ease her mind took patience and answering the same questions repeatedly. Redirecting her worked for a brief while. Mostly TLC gave her the courage to get past the worry and fretting so she could relax.

7.

A Wanderer Or An Explorer

Wanderer. The label was given to a thin, squeaky voiced lady named Sara. Maybe it's time to come up with some new terms. Not long ago I heard the term explorer. Now if it was someone who wanders often like Sara, we could say she was a constant explorer. Don't you think Sara would have liked that term better when we are speaking about her?

She spent most of her day in the care center following the aides around. We'd go into a resident's room with Sara right behind us. We closed the door before she could follow us in, expecting to have privacy. She'd open the door and peek in to see what we were doing only to be told she'd have to wait in the hall until we came back out.

"I want to come in, too," Sara complained in a plaintive voice.

"You can't. We're helping a man in here," I explained through the crack in the door, thinking she'd want no part of that."

"What's the difference?" Sara snapped at me.

What made her so bold to think she could come in while we were assisting a man who was a stranger to her? It was because of Alzheimer's disease. Her inhibition/impulse control was affected by Alzheimer's. That caused her to use bad judgment to enter a room where she shouldn't be. That was our explanation at the time.

There's more to it than that. Understanding why they do the things they do is a good reason to know as much as we can about their lives. We learned much more about why this lady didn't mind entering a man's room after we did our homework about her past. Sara had been an emergency room nurse during her working years. Instinct told her she was our supervisor, and she should be keeping an eye on us while we cared for a patient. Sara wanted to make sure we did a good job, because she was concerned about the patient's health. Knowing that information changed our way of thinking completely.

Patiently, we redirected Sara from the room, and tried to defuse the annoyance she felt at us for not letting her come in a room with us. While we were at it, we now understood why she followed us all the time. Even though she had no memory of her days as a nurse, she felt she belonged to the nursing staff at the facility so she was content with her surroundings.

Once I knew about Sara's past, I understood other things she did. Often Sara would walk over to a resident in a wheelchair, bend over and ask kindly, "How are you today?" Then she'd give that person a compassionate pat on the shoulder or hand before she moved on. Alzheimer's disease had stolen her memory of the past, but it could never remove the compassion in her soul which had made her a good nurse. She still felt like a caregiver. Somehow watching Sara made me feel that those of us who are a caregiver always keep our caregiver's heart if we get Alzheimer's. In her confused world, she lost the ability to do her job, but she kept busy comforting others. There was no way she could do that job wrong, and it gave her some comfort and a sense of satisfaction.

There was another time when the nurse in Sara showed itself.

The charge nurse wanted Sara to take her pills. Sara refused. They had some discussion about the matter which upset Sara. She walked toward me with the nurse following behind her. The angry woman wanted me to protect her since she thought of me as her friend.

"Make her go away," Sara growled.

"What's the matter?"

"She won't leave me along! Make her go away."

"I want Sara to take her meds," the nurse said. "See if you can get her to."

I put my arm around Sara's shoulders to show her I was on her side and looked her in the eyes. "Sara, the nurse wants to give you some medicine to make you feel better. Please, will you take it for me?"

"Okay," Sara relented, turning to the nurse. "Give me your old medicine."

"Oh good! You're going to take the pills?" The nurse asked.

"No, I'm not," Sara said. Then nodding in my direction, she said, "If she wants them so bad, I'm going to stick them up her butt."

"Oh no! Don't give Sara those pills yet," I said, beginning to back up. "Until I get away from here."

So much for trying to convince Sara that I was her friend. Paranoia helped her decide I was siding with the nurse against her. To my surprise, she seemed to remember more about being a nurse than I thought she did. I wasn't sticking around to see if she was going to make good on her threat.

Sometimes when a person is restless, they need a simple task to do. Not everyone makes a task for themselves like Sara did when she consoled the other residents. Perhaps a simple task could be folding towels and wash cloths or dusting furniture. Those are tasks a person could do until she becomes bored or tired. Just unfold the towels when you get out of the person's sight so she can start over.

After she has rubbed the coffee table with a dusting cloth, to keep her dignity in tact, don't say the furniture is polished until it glows so she should stop now. Just let her enjoy doing a productive job that she can succeed at. When she thinks the job is done, praise her for helping and for doing a good job. That means so much to her self esteem.

My mother had a stroke. She regained the use of her right hand, but she needed to use a walker for balance. Brain damage left her unable to remember how to weave on her rug looms and without the stamina that type of work required. My mother had three looms. Having been a busy, hard working woman all her life, I knew that sitting was not going to be good for her. Developing a feeling of uselessness would cause depression to set in. So I tackled what my mother liked doing best. I learned how to weave rugs. Believe me when I say without Mom being able to teach me, I found out learning how did not come easily. I had not inherited my mother's crafty knack for weaving. Quite frankly, I didn't pay as much attention as I should have when I watched her weave. Always in the back of my mind was the thought that Mom would somehow convince me I should help her. I could always say I didn't know how when the time came.

Well, the time came in a way I hadn't expected with Mom's stroke. All at once I was on my own with no tips from Mom. But I did master the art of weaving and put Mom to work winding the shuttles full of cloth strips for me to put through the warp. She sat beside me while we talked and worked. Mostly I talked. She listened, because the stroke had affected her speech. Besides being good range of motion for her hands and arms, winding the strips on the shuttle made her feel useful. The fact that she was happy doing something she liked to do and was familiar with meant the world to her as well as me. I had succeeded in giving her a purpose to live.

On the other hand, my father, who had Alzheimer's, kept busy as an explorer. He loved being outdoors. Living on an acreage was a good thing for him and a bad thing for Mom and me. He had plenty of room to roam and no neighbors that he could bother, but we had to keep watching him. A busy highway ran in front of the house, an accident waiting to happen if Dad wandered onto it. Cornfields, with corn taller than he was, surrounded the acreage and made for constant worries that he would get lost in the field.

I wanted some warning mechanism to signal Mom and me when Dad went near the outside door. Not some blaring, annoying alarm but something that wouldn't frighten or anger Dad. I found an advertisement in a magazine and ordered a brightly colored, motion detector rooster. Dad was always a farmer at heart. My parents had chickens until he wasn't able to take care of them anymore. That rooster was just what I thought we needed.

Father's day was close when the rooster came. I needed a reason to give Dad the rooster without him suspecting why so I gave it to him as a gift. When he unwrapped the rooster, he looked it over. The look on his face said what kind of gift is this, but he just said, "Thank you, Sister." Talking fast, I explained that I knew how much he liked chickens, and when I saw that rooster I thought he might like it. I said I knew the perfect place to set his rooster. Dad followed me out on the back porch. I placed the rooster on a small table by the door.

"There now, Dad. That rooster looks pretty good setting there, doesn't he?"

Dad nodded agreeably, but I had the feeling the reason he liked the rooster there was the fact the back porch was as far away from his chair as that rooster could possibly get. That rooster, with his neck stretched out and his breast puffed up, crow three times whenever anyone moved in front of his motion detector eye on his breast.

28

When Dad past by on his way outside, the rooster crowed. My father didn't pay any attention, but we were alerted. I gave myself an imaginary pat on the back for a brilliant solution.

Of course with so many windows on the porch, the rooster crowed at every sparrow that flew by. As Mom became tired and frustrated as a caregiver, she grew annoyed by the rooster's constant crowing. Probably because she had to check to see if Dad left the house more often than she needed to.

Eventually when I came to visit, I would find the rooster with his back to the door. That didn't do us much good when we need to know Dad's where abouts. The rooster crowed at a lilac branch swinging in the breeze or a bird in flight right outside the window. However with quiet patience, I was determined to use the rooster for the purpose I gave him to Dad. I turned that chicken around to face the door while I was at my parents. Mom turned his back to the door as soon as I left. Somehow in-between that chicken's rotation, we managed to keep an eye on Dad.

When my father became so disoriented trying to find the bathroom in the night, he went outside. Mom was so tired that she no longer woke up when he got out of bed. Cool temperatures had set in that fall, and there was Dad outside in just his pajama top. He did that while my son was visiting. Thank goodness, Duane heard my father cough and knew he was exploring.

This was a new experience for my son as he asked my father why he was outside.

Dad said, "I was looking for the bathroom." He had his back to the outside door. Just as soon as he walked out into the darkness, he was lost. He said to Duane, "It's cold out here."

As he lead his grandfather back inside, Duane replied, "You might not be so cold if you left your pajamas on."

Since Dad still remembered how to turn the knob that unlocked the door, we decided to buy double locks. My older brother, Bill, installed the locks. Mom locked the door and hid the key so Dad couldn't use it. But since Mom had a tendency to forget where she hid the key or if some unforeseen problem came up, my brother and I had keys made so we could get into the house.

I often tell caregivers about this experience. People with dementia wander away and get lost all the time. What I always hear is, "He never does that." Believe me at some point in the progression of the disease he or she will. We never expected Dad to unlock the door and leave the house in the middle of the night. It happened.

8.

Being Repetitive

Repetitive behaviors can be physical or verbal. Someone with Alzheimer's disease may tear paper into tiny pieces, rummage through drawers often, or make a motion in the air like they are dusting furniture to name a few.

That's the need of people to be busy. Whether it be a housewife or someone who left the house to work every day, they had a busy productive life until Alzheimer's took over. A part of them still feels they have work to do even if it is tearing paper into tiny pieces.

Find someone rummaging through drawers or the contents of those drawers are dumped in a heap on the bed. A caregiver might think what a mess. People with Alzheimer's loses items easily. That's because they hide the items in places less obvious than that drawer. Besides in the time it takes them to search, they forget what they were hunting. If they don't fretting really sets in when the item stays lost. Most of the time, the item is something that has meant a lot to that person. Perhaps a wallet or purse. Buy a few more at garage sales and keep handy. Get one out of your stash and exclaim that you found it for the person.

Then there is the meticulous housekeeper or man that likes everything in it's place. In the middle stage of Alzheimer's, those people may be dusting in mid air. Try giving them a dust rag and see what happens. Because everything has to be tidy, someone might try picking up a bit of lint or scarp of paper off the floor and fall. When an obsessive nature takes over, nothing in the house looks clean enough. I've seen the chrome wore off the sink faucets by repeated rubbing to clean them. Maybe polishing silverware might be more constructive.

Often, the repetitive behavior is verbal. The same question is repeated over and over, but the person doesn't remember that he/she has said the same thing before. Maybe what the person is asking isn't what he really wants to know. There is an underlying cause for the thought that's stuck in that person's mind. We need to look for it to help make the person less anxious.

The following are examples of questions frequently asked.

"When do we eat?"

That could mean the person is hungry. Try giving a snack to see if it helps. Most of the time a person with Alzheimer's has a very poor appetite. Sometimes they don't remember the last meal. Sometimes they leave the table before they finish eating. So they should be hungry.

Why do they leave the table too soon? It might be that the person doesn't realize they need to eat to live. Maybe it's the over stimulation of so many people in a nursing home dining room and so much noise coming from every direction. Voices, silverware clinking against china and helpers moving about can make for a confusing situation that the person with Alzheimer's wants to get away from as quick as he can even it that means going hungry. Extra snacks and nutritional, finger foods that the person can eat on the go might help. At home, the confusing situation might be a family dinner, a television or radio in the background.

Let me tell you about one lady who never remembered her mealtime experiences. One day I was walking with ex-nurse, Sara. She turned and asked softly, "Have you had lunch yet?"

"Yes, I've eaten," I replied.

"What did you have?"

"Fried potatoes and a hamburger."

Sara turned to face me, looking hurt. "Why didn't you call me when it was time to eat? I didn't get anything to eat today for lunch."

I said I was sorry to hear that. I knew she'd been served lunch and had forgotten. I offered to go get her something to eat right away.

I fell into that one, didn't I? Sara couldn't remember that she had lunch. She was hurt because she thought I forgot to let her know when I ate. However, she often got up from the table in the middle of her meal and wandered off. Excuse me, I meant she went exploring.

Naturally, she would be hungry later on. Sometimes she ate better if we handed her something she could eat whenever she wanted it. Snacks in her walker bag were a great discovery when she finally did sit down to rest. Thin, weary Sara needed every morsel of food she was willing to eat even if she didn't remember the snack or meal later on.

Another question is, "When is my son coming to visit?"

Being forewarned made the person anxious about the son's arrival. Sometimes it is better to not mention a visit or a doctor appointment until the time comes. Anticipation and restless worry about what is going to happen keeps the person on edge. Maybe they remember enough to know what is going to happen that day, but not when. Or maybe they know something is going to happen and not what. Something in their mind triggers worry, because they know an event is about to happen. Since they can't remember exact details, they fear they might make a mistake.

Another question. "What time is it?"

The same question can be repeated over and over and becomes annoying to a stressed caregiver. Answering the question truthfully will do no good if the first answer wasn't enough. Try to get the person's mind on another subject. The problem may be as simple as the person is bored. Remember he can't process that he has asked for the time of day repeatedly. Think of his brain as a computer that is fully loaded. That brain can't take in any more new information. Therefore, the answer as well as the question bounces away.

If changing the subject didn't help, try giving that person a task to do to get his mind off the question. Everyone needs to be needed and helpful. Someone with Alzheimer's feels helpless and confused all the time. It's a good feeling to be able to do something helpful for the caregiver. Just remember not to criticize the finished effort, because whatever the task is, it won't be done just as you would like it. Praise, praise and more praise will make that person's day.

For someone in the first stage of Alzheimer's a caregiver might try writing down the time of an appointment and a meal. Have the person carry it in his pocket or place the note on the refrigerator. Somewhere that the person might be able to check each time he becomes apprehensive. Expect there to come a time when the person will forget to look for the note then the caregiver is back to square one. The time comes when the person with AD doesn't remember he has an appointment. You show up to take him to the doctor. He is surprised and upset. It's all your fault for not telling him about the doctor visit. Go along with him. He's right. You are wrong. You say you forgot to tell him, but you'll help him get ready. That makes it all right in his mind. He didn't forget. You did.

Another example of repetition is a friendly lady with a wide smile who had a fascination with numbers. At times, Lois started a conversation with the aides by blurting out a number. During the shift, she'd continue to repeat that number and others over again to get our attention. We tried to change the subject, but Lois didn't want any part of that. She'd go right back to saying numbers.

After Lois passed away, I went to her visitation to extend my sympathies to the family. One of her daughters showed me, she had purchased a bingo card and marker to put in the casket with Lois. Until then I didn't know that she had been an avid bingo player.

It was as if a light bulb went off in my head when I thought of all the times Lois repeatedly called out numbers. I asked the daughter if Lois could have been playing bingo. She didn't think so since some of the numbers Lois called were higher than bingo numbers, but it's very possible that Lois had forgotten how high the bingo numbers go. When the aides couldn't get her mind off calling a number, they would say another number. This became a game to Lois as she'd always say a number higher than the one we called, and wait for our reply with a grin that said she was having fun. That's maybe why sometimes the numbers grew larger. All that time, we were playing bingo with Lois and didn't know it. But the smile on her face showed how much fun she had at her imaginary bingo game. Imagine, we made that woman's life happier and didn't understand why. We didn't do our homework with this woman's history, but we lucked out.

Remember if a person repeatedly tries to leave the building at the same time of day that might be when he went to work, or she went to pick up the children at school. If a resident tries to get into the nursing home kitchen, she may have been a cook or just wants to fix a meal for her family.

These repetitions are a good reason to find out as much as you can about the persons you will be taking care of. Relatives can tell you things that will work to soothe restlessness, trigger a memory or in some way make the repetitive things the person with Alzheimer's does easier for the caregiver to understand.

9.

Carrie's Angels

Faith can sustain people with dementia to the very end. That was what happened to Carrie.

When she entered the care center with only a few days left to live, Carrie was very pale, gaunt, weak and experiencing intermittent waves of pain. She didn't look much like the pretty, tall, slender, elegant dresser that I remembered from the past.

I helped her with her first evening meal, because Carrie was too weak to feed herself. Since she didn't have an appetite, it was a challenge to get her to nibble at the food on her plate.

Suddenly, Carrie grimaced as pain seared through her body. She cried out, "Why is the Lord putting me through all this?"

I didn't answer her, because I didn't know what to say. I took her hand and held it tightly until the pain passed. I hoped the feel of her hand in mine might help her to know that she wasn't alone.

In a few minutes, Carrie relaxed as the pain went away.

She opened her eyes. Looking around the room, she tried to place where she was, and hoped to see something that looked familiar to her.

"What is that?" Carrie asked with her eyes directed at the small chest at the foot of her bed.

"It's an angel." I walked over and picked up the 4 inch tall, white angel with wings stretched out as if she was ready to take flight. With Carrie's dimming eyesight, the angel must have been a small, white blur from where she laid.

I held the angel directly in front of Carrie so she could see it. With her eyes focused on the angel, her face took on a peaceful look. I placed the angel behind the plate of food and encouraged Carrie to continue to eat. She managed to get a few more bites down. All the while, she kept her eyes glued to the miniature angel.

The exertion of eating soon wore Carrie out. She closed her eyes, laid her head on the pillow, and steeled herself for another wave of pain. I saw it coming this time. I wanted to help her get through the moment so I picked up the angel, placed it in the palm of Carrie's left hand and closed her slim fingers around it.

"Hold onto the angel, Carrie. Maybe that will help," I said.

That evening Carrie's husband and son came to see her. They hadn't been in her room long before the son stepped out in the hall and stopped me. He sounded upset as he asked me, "Have you seen a small, white angel in my mother's room? It's missing."

"Sure. I gave it to your mother to hold earlier. Did you look in the bed by her?"

"No, I'll look there," he said.

Later when I had a moment, I stopped to check on Carrie. Her husband and son were quietly standing by her bed, watching her sleep.

"Find the angel?" I asked softly.

"No, I didn't," the son said sadly.

I bent over the bed to speak in Carrie's ear. "Carrie, your son wants to see the angel. I'm going to lift your hand and see if it's there."

I picked up her limp hand, spread open on the bed beside her and uncovered the angel. Handing it to her son, I explained that I gave it to her because it had given Carrie comfort to hold the angel when she was in pain.

"I'm so glad that you did that for my mother. The angel means a lot to her. I was worried that it had gotten lost," he said. Relief covered his face. "My mother went to church every Sunday and taught Sunday school for years. Her faith has sustained her through this illness. I want to hang this angel on a string from the ceiling so it dangles at the foot of her bed where she can see it."

"That's a great idea," I said. It was plain to see he wanted to do something to comfort his mother. Hanging up the angel for her would comfort him, too. Still, I couldn't let go of the idea that Carrie couldn't see that small angel flying above her. She needed to have one closer. So I explained, "She took such comfort from holding the angel, but since it's breakable, it probably wasn't a good idea to have it in bed with her. I wonder if you could find one of those cloth angels. She could hold that in her hands."

The son's eyes lit up at the prospect of doing something to help his mother. "I'll have it here by tomorrow," he vowed.

The next afternoon when I entered Carrie's room, I immediately noticed the peaceful look on her face and the reason why. Squeezed tightly in her hands was a muslin angel who's full skirt was draped over Carrie's chest.

When Carrie began to decline that day, her grip on the angel relaxed. The angel would fall beside her. Each time the aides checked on her, they placed the angel on her chest and curled her fingers around it. That night Carrie passed away with the muslin angel in her hands, and the tiny, ceramic angel hovering above her bed to guide her on her final journey.

Whether it be holding an angel, a bible that the resident can no longer read, or a rosary that has always been an important solace, as the resident's caregiver, care enough to give the resident that comfort.

God will give his angel charge of you to guard you in all your ways.

-- Psalm 91:11 - 13

10.

Job Motivation

Ella, a shadow of her former self, moved quickly through the halls. Her passion was the kitchen which she tried to enter often. When she did, immediately a cook would escort her back out.

Signs were posted on the doors. "Do not enter, Ella". The thought was that Ella would read the signs and stay away from the kitchen, but Ella had her own ideas about those signs. I came up behind her one night as she peered closely at the sign on the kitchen door. Raising the pen she held in her hand, Ella began to mark over her name on the sign.

In a low voice, I said, "No, no, Ella."

At the sound of my voice, Ella took off down the hall without looking back. She knew she had been caught.

So why did Ella have such a passion for invading the kitchen? She had been a dietitian in a large hospital for years. She still felt the need to work as a dietitian even though she didn't understand what the job was all about anymore.

Going to work had been the central part of this lady's life for years. She still felt the need to stay busy, and she wanted it to be in the surroundings that she was familiar with -- the kitchen. So the kitchen supervisor gave Ella a clipboard with a monthly menu on it. At meal times, she followed the person who set the tables, carrying her clipboard. Once, Ella gave a young man, setting the tables, a promotion to the fifth floor and a raise. The care center is all on one floor, but Ella didn't know that. In her mind as happens to people with Alzheimer's, she had gone back in her past and still worked in a large, multi floor hospital. We smiled when her evaluations of the meals weren't always complimentary once we figured out the evaluations depended on whether she liked the food that was served to her.

When we gave Ella the clipboard and let her supervise the dining room it made her feel useful again and content because she was busy. At the same time, we had cared enough to find a solution for Ella's invasions of the kitchen so she wouldn't have to be upset. We realized why she wanted to be there in the first place. She wanted to work. Everyone has the need to be busy so we should find something for them to do whether it be a made up job of folding laundry, a gadget to inspect or a photo or memory box for that person to sort through.

We posted other signs for Ella, plus the ones on the kitchen and exit doors. One evening, I saw Ella turning down the covers on a bed across the hall from her room. I told her to come with me, and I'd show her where her bed was.
    "Look at the sign on the door. It says, "Ella's room"," I pointed out. "Look at the sign on your closet. It says, "Ella's closet", and the one over your bed says, "Ella's bed". The room you was in wasn't yours."
    "I know that," Ella told me. Then she paused to think about how she was going to explain her actions. She gave me an authoritative look of someone who was used to taking charge. "But if I was in the wrong room, I had a perfectly good

reason to be there." Again she paused, looking puzzled that time, before she continued, "I just can't think of what it is for the moment."

Then one evening it was clear we'd have to take her signs down. I watched as Ella went down the wrong hall. She stood on tiptoes to read the name plates beside each room's door. She disappeared into one of the rooms, and I suspected that she was going to get ready for bed so I followed her.

I was right. The little lady was turning down the covers on a bed. "What are you doing, Ella?"

"I'm getting ready for bed."

"This isn't your room. Didn't you see the name on the sign outside wasn't yours?"

"Yes, I saw that, but there are so many signs around here with my name on them that I didn't know which door to go in so I decided to pick one that didn't have my name on it."

You know that statement made sense to me. People who have Alzheimer's disease reach a point where they can still read, but they can't comprehend what the words mean. Ella may have misunderstood the line "Do not enter" on each sign and thought having her name on it gave her permission to enter the door the sign was on. No wonder she was confused, because each time she tried to go in a door with the sign on it, we kept telling her even though her name was on the sign she couldn't enter the room. What so often happens with Alzheimer's disease is that reasoning powers go awry. Ella reasoned why not pick a room that didn't have a sign posted with her name on it. Maybe we would leave her alone. Of course, that didn't happen.

11.

Your Treasures Are Mine

One day former nurse, Sara, came to meet me as if she was a lady on a mission. Her heavy, white, knit sweater tail was rolled up and gripped tightly in both hands. She couldn't remember one CNA from another, but Sara always seemed to pick me when she wanted to talk.

She scooted her feet in short, choppy steps as if she meant business as she came toward me.

"Hello, Sara," I greeted, smiling at her.

"Where have you been?" She snapped at me in her supervisor tone.

"I just got here," I explained, feeling like I was already in trouble for something, but I didn't know what.

"Well, I've been looking for you all day!" Her voice rose in annoyance.

"I'm here now so what can I do for you?"

"I have something to give you to take to my room." Sara unrolled her sweater and handed me a remote control.

Swell, I'm thinking. This is a facility full of televisions so it's going to take a while to figure out which resident owned

44

the remote.

Why did Sara trust me with her treasure? Simple. She couldn't find her room, and she was getting tired of carrying the remote hidden in her sweater. She had a feeling that no one else should see it until she got it to her room. Should I have tried to tell her that it was wrong to take someone else's property? Or that there was no way that I was going to take someone else's remote to her room? The answer is no.

Before she had Alzheimer's disease, Sara lived alone in her home for some time. Her house was her domain, and the objects in that home were hers. No one in that house said, "Put that back. It's not yours." Now she thought the care center she lived in was her home -- every room in it. So in her mind she should have been able to pick up and carry with her whatever treasures were laying about.

The feeling of displacement from familiar surroundings was frightening enough so why should we make it worse by telling Sara she did the wrong thing. Can you imagine you are living in a home that has suddenly grown in room size and not one of the rooms looks familiar to you? But the advantage in Sara's mind was that she had so many interesting treasures in this home to look at and carry around. She saw nothing wrong with wanting to move each of the items to different places in that large house.

12.

Nap Time

As CNAs know, the trouble with being on your feet all day, walking from one end of a nursing home to the other, is that your legs get tired as well as the rest of your body. Add to that the fact that the person doing the walking is 90 years old. That person really gets tired.

The aides knew it was time for Mable to take an afternoon nap long before she was ready to give in to lying down. Taking turns walking with Mable to her room, her caregivers helped her get her feet on the bed, covered her up and left the room. A few feet down the hall, we'd hear the shuffle of her short, choppy steps, look back and there was Mable gaining on us. The time we spent trying to get her to lie down was wasted. Her attitude became more cranky with each trip back to her room until finally she refused to go with us. All the while, Mable was slowing down from hours of roaming the halls. We worried that she would fall.

One afternoon, I took Mable by the hand and asked her to come for a walk with me. Of course, we ended up in her room. I sat her down on the bed, helped her get her feet up, covered her up and left the room just as we had done every other day. And like every other day, I looked back to find Mable right behind me.

Again, I took her back to her room to repeat putting her in bed. "You need to lie down for a nap. Aren't you tired?"

"Yes," she admitted.

"Well, why won't you stay in bed then and take a nap?"

"Because I want you to stay here with me." Mable's plaintive voice held an unspoken plea.

There we had it. She was lonely and fearful of being left in that empty room by herself. Add to that the fact, she was in a large place where the sounds of doors banging, lights going off, a variety of strange voices, and loud alarms seemed endless. In her confusion, she feared everything around her and what she heard. Now I understood why Mable kept following us out of the room.

What did I do? I promised that I'd stay with her. I pulled up a chair, sat down by her bed and held her hand. Fighting sleep for a few minutes, Mable peeked over at me from narrowed eyelids to make sure I was still there until finally her hand went limp in mine, and she breathed deeply in a sound sleep. Then I slipped out of the room.

Taking the time to sit by her bedside to give Mable the peace of mind that it took to get her to rest took far less time than walking her back to her room on those repeated trips. When she woke up rested and ready for the evening meal, Mable wasn't upset that I hadn't stayed with her during the nap, because she had Alzheimer's disease. She didn't remember that I'd promised to stay.

13.

The Escapee

The front door alarm sounded, blaring through the facility. Each resident with dementia has a code alert bracelet that sets the alarm off so we know when they go outside by themselves. As usual, the aides ran to see who was escaping.

"It's Martha. There she goes across the sun room now, headed for the outside door," an aide said as she rushed to stopped the "runaway" resident.

"That's the third time she's been out that door today. All we get done is run after her," complained another aide. "I better go with you. It might take two of us to talk her back in this time. She didn't want to come back very bad the last time."

The two aides entered the sun room just as Martha reached the outside door. "Wait up. We want to talk to you, Martha," one of the aides called to her.

Martha, a disgruntled look on her face, turned her walker around and stood still, waiting for the aides to catch up. Her slim, tall frame was braced in a defiant stance as she felt the bright sun's inviting warmth caress her back.

"What do you want now?" She snapped.

"We want to walk back with you," one of the aides said,

motioning toward the inside door.

"Why?"

"You shouldn't go outside now."

"Oh, I know I'm not supposed to go outside by myself. It's either too hot, too windy, getting ready to rain or something else. I've heard it all so what is it now?" She complained as she made a half turn to look longingly through the glass door.

"Supper is ready so you should come back in and eat while the food is hot."

Begrudgingly, Martha came back with the aides, only to try to leave again whenever she went by the front door. She couldn't understand why she couldn't go outside alone anymore. Alzheimer's disease kept Martha from realizing that she wouldn't know how to get back in the building even if she was standing near the door. She didn't have the ability to reason that if she walked too far away, she might be too tired to make it back to the care center on her own or that she'd get lost.

For her it was frustrating to be told she couldn't go for a walk alone. Martha had always been able to come and go as she pleased. She didn't like people telling her she couldn't go outside when she wanted to enjoy a lovely, summer day.

Martha's daughter was informed that her mother kept trying to leave the building. The daughter said she understood what the problem was, and she shared the reason with us. For years, Martha had gone for long walks. She loved to be outside and knew that walking exercise was good for her. Martha wasn't trying to escape, but she simply wasn't ready to give up her walks.

The solution was simple. Find someone who could go for a walk with Martha, then maybe she'd be willing to stay in the building after the walk. When winter set in, we'd have to come up with a plan to keep Martha from going outside. The fact that it was too cold to go outside wouldn't mean anything to her, and she remembered all the other excuses we'd used. She didn't want to hear them again. So we asked her daughter if she could write a few notes to her mother and leave them with us. When Martha grew restless we would tell her that the mail came, and she had a letter from her daughter. She needed to come back inside to read it. By the time, Martha finished the letter we hoped that she would forget she intended to take a walk for that moment anyway.

Many times, the reason a person might try eloping is they think they need to go to work. Watch the time of day they head for the door and find out if that might be when they left home for work or to pick up the children from school. A quick distraction will usually work each time. Just a few minutes away from the door will give them time to forget they wanted to leave.

My father leaving the house was one of the challenges of taking care of him for my mother and me. As a farmer, he loved the outdoors and working the land. Once he retired from running a gas station, he spent much of his daylight hours in the garden. The soil was so cultivated that when Mom and I went to pick peas or green beans, we sank into the soft dirt. There was no getting Dad to rest. Finally, he got heat exhaustion from being in the hot sun too long and that lessened his working hours for quite some time.

As his memory failed and his balance became worse, we had to watch that he didn't fall as he pushed the garden plow across the long garden. With his shuffling gait, he staggered behind the plow, holding on for dear life. At that point, I wasn't sure if he was holding the plow up or if the plow was holding him up.

Back in those days not as much was known by elderly caregivers at home about how to make life easier for someone with Alzheimer's. Though I was learning as much as I could, Mom was in the dark most of the time. What I did comment on or make suggestions to try went in one of her ears and out the other. She didn't see my father as a sick man who couldn't help the odd things he said or did. Mom saw what she wanted to see, the healthy man she married. She didn't want to understand that he was confused and forgetful.

Most days, I went over to my parents early and stayed until time to go to work on second shift at the nursing home. If it was my day off, I stayed all day. One morning, Dad was already in the garden when I came. I watched for a minute as he slowly pushed the plow across the garden then went inside.

"Dad sure looks industrious this morning. He has quite a few rows plowed already," I said.

Mom frowned at me. "You need to go out there and stop him before he tears the whole garden up."

One thing I learned early on was if Mom wanted Dad talked into something she thought he might object to, she'd let me do it. That way he wouldn't be mad at her. That is a good idea. The caregiver has a hard 24/7 job and doesn't need the added stress of making the care receiver mad at her. In Mom's case, she always expected me to be able to talk Dad out of doing something without making him mad. She didn't have that knack.

"Why? He seems to be doing okay," I said, surprised. I thought as long as Dad loved what he was doing, he should do it. Ordinarily Mom would have agreed. Working in the garden kept Dad out of her way.

"You have to stop him now. He just plowed up a whole row of carrots and beets," Mom snapped.

I couldn't help giggling. Dad probably couldn't see well enough to make out the newly sprouted plants. Then again maybe he thought they were weeds, but I had heard him say often enough that he wish beets and carrots had never been invented. He would starve if those two vegetables were the only things in the garden.

Mom glared at me. I stopped giggling and compromised. I reminded her Dad plowing up those two rows was probably no accident. She had plenty of time to replant both vegetables, and I'd go tell Dad to watch carefully where he plowed.

14.

The Social Butterfly

Often a band comes to delight the residents at the care center with the polka music they enjoyed in their past. The residents clap while couples dance to the music in their brightly colored, square dance costumes. As a finale, "Happy Birthday" is played for all the residents who celebrated a birthday that month. Everyone has a good time.

At the end of the evening, the band packs up, and tells everyone good bye as they shake hands with the residents. One of the people they stopped to talk to was Grace. Her happy smile stood out, and her sparkling eyes danced in remembrance of when she was young.

Though she seemed to comprehend what others said to her, Grace answered back with a language of her own -- usually the phrase "If he." For her, those words seemed to fit every occasion, by changing the tone of her voice depending whether Grace was happy or upset.

As the band carried their instruments out the door, Grace followed, beaming her smile at them. Her wheeled walker held at arms length, she swayed from side to side at the hips as she walked, hurrying to keep up with the band members.

We watched her as she neared the door for fear she'd go

outside with the band. Aides took turns trying to talk Grace away from the door which became an irritation to her.

One evening, Grace made it out the door behind the band into the sun room. I tried to get her to come back in, but she elbowed my hand away.

"If he," she said crossly. Then she smiled brightly at the departing guests as she waved. "If he," she called cheerfully after them as if she was trying to say, "I'll see you next time. Come back soon." As the band pulled away, she turned and willingly walk back inside with me.

That's when I realized keeping an eye on Grace was all right, because she might have walked out the door with the band. Though I do believe if that had happened, someone would have realized that Grace wasn't a member of the band and escorted her back in. But we shouldn't have worried so much about her leaving the building that we upset her. If we had been paying attention to what she was doing, we'd have known that Grace was practicing her social graces just like she'd done many times in her home. Dementia may have taken away much from Grace, but how to behave at the end of a social event was still very much a part of her.

15.

Customer Service

If a care center has a warm and friendly atmosphere, then the resident and the family members will adjust easier to the resident living there so TLC from the staff should be applied not only to the residents but their families. We need to realize one of the hardest things in the world for a caregiver to do is relinquish the care of a loved one to strangers in a large facility.

Care centers are looked upon as a place to avoid until someone needs to be admitted to one. On a tour of a care center, first impressions weigh heavily on the family's decision to place a loved one there. The family carries overwhelming feelings of guilt for putting a loved one in a care center so it's up to us to show them how well we will take care of their loved one. Those guilty feelings can even come back to haunt the family when the loved one is gone if they are unhappy with the care the loved one received.

As the time nears for a loved one to depart this world, the family may spend hours sitting by the bedside. As aides, we do what we can to show them we care during this sad time. We want the family to feel they made the right decision to let us take over the care for the loved one.

Once in a while, it's not a whole family by the bedside but one individual. Can you imagine how lonely and sad that must be, sitting alone by the side of a loved one who's dying?

Joe was a devoted son who came every Sunday to visit his mother. Tiny, quiet, sweet Ethel looked forward to those visits. She wasn't much of a conversationalist and probably never had been unless something was important enough to her that she felt it needed to be said. A good percentage of the time, she bowed her head and look piercingly over the top of her glasses as we talked to her, and we'd get a faint smile or a quiet, "Ya."

Her son's devotion carried on to the end. He spent hours by her bedside. Later in the evening when it was my break time, I thought about how Joe must be feeling, sitting alone by his mother's bed with only sad thoughts for company so I decided to spend my break with Joe and his mother.

"Hi, I'm back," I said to Joe. "I'm on break so I wondered if you'd like me to keep you company for a few minutes?"

"That would be great! Have a seat." I heard the relief in his voice. He was glad to have someone join him if only for a short time.

"Ethel isn't doing very well now," I said, trying to prepare him for what was imminent.

"I know she isn't," Joe said sadly.

I knew a story about his mother that I thought Joe might enjoy, and I wondered if it would help him pass the time easier if I talked about her. I respected her for the rugged life she had lived as a devoted farmer's wife and mother. Ethel had made the most of her long life, and I was glad that our paths had crossed. Besides I felt my talking about her as I knew her was better than the two of us sitting in silence, waiting for the end.

The story I told was about Ethel at meal times. She sat,

hands in her lap with her head bent down, with no intention of eating. The aides would feed her a bite or two if we were lucky, then she'd turn her head away and button her lips tightly together. The few bites we did get her to accept, she'd take forever to chew to keep from eating more.

When I scolded her for not eating, Ethel's reply was that she was 93 years old. I told her age didn't make any difference. She still needed to eat no matter how old she was.

We knew that Ethel liked sweets. When our attention was turned to another resident at the table, Ethel would eat her dessert by herself. We tried sitting the dessert bowl out of Ethel's reach to get her to eat the food on her plate first. She would stare at us with that soul searching look over the top of her glasses, then turn her head away when we tried to feed her those distasteful, sugar free vegetables.

Chocolate drops was Ethel's favorite candy. Her daughter brought a pint jar to keep by Ethel's bedside so we could give her a candy kiss when we got her up or before she went to bed.

I decided to try to bribe Ethel to see if she'd eat her meals. Tempting her with dessert hadn't been enough incentive to get her to eat but maybe the chocolate drops would be. Before going down to the assisted dining room, I went to Ethel's room and took three chocolate drops from her jar. With a definite plan in mind, I sat down by Ethel at the table. With deliberation, I placed all three candy kisses in a row above Ethel's plate out of reach I thought.

"Ethel, look what I brought for you -- some of your candy kisses. Would you like to eat them for supper?"

With a suspicious look, Ethel peered at me as she slightly nodded her head. "Ya."

"Great! What I want you to do first before I give you the candy is to eat some of the food on your plate. Maybe it looks like too much to eat so how about I divide each portion of food in half. If you clean up half of each thing on your plate then you get a piece of candy."

56

My plan was to get her to start eating again then maybe we could increase the portions just a little each time until she finally ate most of the meal.

Ethel nodded in agreement, opening her mouth for the first bite of meatloaf. As I promised when she cleaned up half of the meatloaf, I unwrapped a chocolate drop and stuck it in her mouth. A look of pleasure flooded over her face as she enjoyed the candy as it melted in her mouth.

In between giving Ethel a bite, I was helping the lady who sat next to her. While I was busy helping Ethel's table mate, Ethel quite smoothly reached over her plate and snatched a candy kiss. By the time I noticed, she was busy concentrating on getting the foil wrapper off as fast as she could with her arthritic fingers. Too late to stop her then so I let her eat the candy, and as I suspected, the green beans didn't appeal to Ethel anymore. I learned to put the candy out of her reach if I wanted her to hold up to her end of the bargain.

My idea worked though. By the time I left on vacation, Ethel began to eat more with the bribe of candy kisses. When I came back to work one of the aides told me the first night I was gone, she fed Ethel, and she forgot to go get the candy kisses. Rather than go after the candy, she decided to see if Ethel would eat without being bribed that one time.

Ethel did eat everything on her plate, and the aide praised her. "Good job, Ethel."

In response, Ethel gave her one of those piercing looks that she used so effectively over the rim of her glasses and declared, "You forgot my three pieces of chocolate!"

Good for Ethel, I thought for speaking up for herself. She had eaten her meal, and she knew she deserved her treat. "Well, did you go get her the candy?" I asked afraid if the aide hadn't that we'd have to start working with Ethel all over again to get her to eat.

"Yes, I did," answered the aide.

That's what I wanted to hear. Ethel needed to know that she could trust us to keep our end of the bargain so she would continue eating.

Her son appreciated the story. He could relate to Ethel's quiet determination when she wanted something.

By then my break was over so I went back to work, but Joe didn't have to stay alone in the room much longer. He caught up with me at the nurse's station and asked me to get the nurse for him. His mother had passed away.

It was a good feeling to know that I helped Joe take his mind off his lonely vigil for that short 15 minutes. He left the nursing home with a good feeling about the care his mother was given and the caregivers he intrusted to take care of a special person in his life. I hoped just maybe near the end if Ethel could hear my voice as I talked about her favorite candy that she was comforted, too.

16.

The Road Map

After a few days off with a bout of stomach flu, I returned to work at the nursing home to find a few cases lingering among the residents. I'll never forget the bad effect my presence had on Lois who had the flu the day of my return.

Another aide and I went to Lois's room to wake her up before the evening meal. I was standing over Lois, patting her on the shoulder and softly saying her name so I wouldn't scare her.

Lois opened her eyes, looked at me and began to cry uncontrollably.

"What's wrong, Lois?"

"I've passed on and gone to Hell!" she sobbed.

I knew I didn't look my best after two days of suffering with the same thing she had now, but I was surprised by her reaction at seeing me.

"No, you haven't passed on. You have the flu, Lois."

"No, no, I know I've passed on, and I'm in Hell," she moaned. "How am I ever going to get back to Elberon?"

I could see that I wasn't going to be able to convince

Lois that she hadn't died so I said, "I don't have a road map, Lois, so which side of Hell is Elberon on?"

She stopped crying to think about that, and I left the room. The next time that Lois needed to be checked, another aide went to see about her. I didn't want to take a chance of upsetting her by associating me with Hell again.

The best thing to do is switch caregivers while a person with dementia is upset with you. After a while, all memory of that moment was gone, and Lois no longer thought of Hell when she saw me.

Please don't take a person with Alzheimer's disease being upset with you personally. The disease destroys the reasoning powers in their brain. Find someone else to take care of the person for awhile and get out of sight. Keep in mind the way that person is feeling won't last long. Whatever triggered the fear, frustration and anger will soon be forgotten.

It's good to keep a sense of humor when working with people with dementia. They lose the knowledge they once had about what is proper to say and what isn't. They can be very uncomplimentary about such things as your hairdo, manner of dress, the size of people, or their looks. Especially as I learned from experience if the person with Alzheimer's thinks that person is related to the devil.

17.

The Greatest Bath

Opal worried about what the care center would be like when she first moved in. She looked for things to like about the place, and the one and only thing she decided was the best care center feature was the bathtub. In her piercingly sharp voice, she stated that the best bath she ever had was in our whirlpool tub. Knowing that it was bath day, and she had something she liked to look forward to did help to brighten her day.

One day, we were talking while I helped Opal with her bath. She said there was one other bath that she had really liked which was a bubble bath she had at one of her granddaughters. Remembering it wistfully, she stated that she'd never get another one like that.

It was close to Christmas so when the staff drew resident names I saw to it that I got her name, because I knew what to get Opal -- a big bottle of Peach bubble bath.

After Christmas day, Opal could hardly wait for her next bath. She settled into the tub while I poured a generous helping of bubble bath oil into the water and turned on the jets. We both watched as the water swirled into millions of tiny, shiny bubbles that rose airily up around Opal.

"Oh, this is nice! Look at all these soft bubbles," she exclaimed.

"That little dab of oil I poured into the water really made a lot of bubbles," I said.

"I'll say! I wish we could take my picture with all these bubbles around me," Opal joked, up to her chin in suds.

Just then an aide came in, watched Opal enjoying her bubble bath and realized that was the happiest she had seen the little woman since she had been admitted to the nursing home. The aide told me not to drain the bathtub until she could bring back the director of nursing. No problem there. Opal was in no hurry to give up her bath.

In no time they were back, and the DON said it looked like Opal was having a great bath.

"Opal says she wishes she could have her picture taken in all these bubbles," I offered, grinning.

"Shall I go get the camera?" Asked the aide.

"No, no, no, I don't want that," Opal stuttered as she chuckled. "I was just kidding."

Once the other aides realized how much pleasure Opal got out of having her bubble bath, they took turns bringing in sweet smelling bottles to keep her in bubbles. Such a simple and what seemed like a small thing at the time, but we gave Opal something to look forward to in a strange place, and she was always ready for her bath.

Bath time is fearful for most people with Alzheimer's disease. When their memory was good, they used a bathtub. Then when their balance wasn't good, they feared falling in the tub or had trouble getting out of it because of arthritis. So they bathed at the sink. Soon the memory of using a bathtub faded. When residents enter the nursing home, they are introduced to a huge bathtub, undressed in front of a stranger, strapped on a cold seat and lifted up in the air then plunked down to the bottom of the bathtub. The door bangs shut. The water gushes at them and rises around them. They can't be sure where the water lever is going to stop. They fear drowning. Is it no wonder they become combative? They're fighting for their life. That feeling is never going to go away, because no matter what you say to the resident you can't rationalize their fear or reason it away.

Most often, it's less fearful for the resident to take a shower. Still the dread of undressing and being hosed down is not a pleasant experience. I try not telling the resident where we are headed until we get there. Keeps them from worrying and resisting. But if that doesn't work, look for another answer that is more agreeable to the resident. Sometimes, I'll ask the resident to take a walk with me which happens to end up in the shower room.

Another example to make life in a care center less frustrating for a resident is this story.

Former school teacher Martha, the lady who liked to walk, had another problem that worried her. As with most people in her generation, Martha didn't always change her clothes every day when she lived at home. In her youth, people may not have possessed many clothes and couldn't afford to buy new wardrobes very often. We need to realize how lucky we are to have all the luxury and conveniences that we do today.

Years ago washing clothes was a dreaded, laborious chore especially if Mom had a large family, as she went from using a scrub board to a wringer washing machine. Think how different we have it now. We throw our laundry in an automatic washer, let it do the work and come back later to put the load in the dryer.

So Martha took her clothes off at night and laid them neatly on her recliner or walker, expecting to be able to put them back on in the morning. The next morning her clothes would be gone, and she'd have to hunt clean clothes out of the closet. This was very frustrating to her.

Often when I'd help her get ready for bed, Martha would ask me not to take her clothes. Of course after the lights were out, I'd grab her neatly folded pile of clothes and hurry out the door before she caught me.

One evening, I slipped in to check on Martha after she had been in bed awhile and noticed her slacks stretched across her walker with a note attached. I unpinned the note and took it into the bathroom to read.

"No, no mercy on the mercy. Very little bit of crisp bandage and no new hard. No dragging. Please leave pants here. --- please leave pants here."

I felt the frustration in that note, written to the thief who continually slipped into Martha's room in the night and stole her clothes. The solution seemed so simple. Replace the clothes on the walker with a clean outfit while Martha was sleeping. By morning, because she had Alzheimer's she wouldn't remember what she wore the day before. She'd start the day less anxious. Maybe that would make the rest of her day go better.

By the way, I repined the note to the clean slacks just in case Martha remembered leaving it.

18.

The Packed Suitcase

For most people, coming to live in the care center is a hard adjustment to make and especially for someone with Alzheimer's disease. They want to go home, but we are never sure at different times which home they mean; a childhood home, the home they raised their family in or their last home -- the retirement apartment. Until they get adjusted, we realize they may try to leave the building at anytime.

Emma hadn't been with us very long when I came out of a room to see the back of her short framed body headed down the hall, carrying a suitcase that was about half the size of her. First of all, it hadn't been a wise thing to leave the suitcase in her room. It reminded her that she could put her possessions back in that suitcase as easily as we had taken them out.

Catching up with her, I asked. "Where are you headed, Emma?"

"I'm going home tonight," she explained.

"Why not wait until morning?" I reasoned as I tagged along. "You have the room paid for."

That reasoning always seems to work on hard working people that were penny savers whether it be a trip to the beauty shop, supper or spending the night. Just tell them the bill has already been paid by someone, and they would be wasting money if they didn't take advantage of whatever service it was.

"Can't do that. I have a driver coming for me, and he'll be waiting for me at the door." Emma kept moving as she talked.

Whoops! The already paid for idea didn't work! Quick thinking time. "Emma, I'm sorry I forgot to tell you the driver called. He wanted us to let you know he had car trouble. He won't be able to come pick you up until morning."

"Really?" She asked in an incredulous tone, stopping to look at me.

"Yes, so why don't you let me carry the suitcase back to your room for you, and I'll help you get ready for bed."

"Okay," she said as she willingly handed me the suitcase.

I put the suitcase back in Emma's closet without looking in it. I thought if I tried to unpack it right then Emma would get upset with me and refuse to go to bed.

A few days later, Emma told me, "I'm not so sure I like living in this place."

"Why not?"

"I don't like to always have to live out of a suitcase."

It was then that I remember that I hadn't looked in her suitcase. So while Emma was out of the room for the evening meal, I took it from the closet and opened it. Inside I found what Emma had decided to leave with. The suitcase held the contents of her underwear drawer, plus a comb, makeup, perfume and lotion from the top drawer. This time, I unpacked the suitcase and took it with me to the basement.

My idea was out of sight out of mind. Emma would entertain enough thoughts of leaving without the reminder of that suitcase. I hoped that it being gone was one less hint.

66

19.

Someone Stole My Pickup

Sometimes saying one thing to a resident leads that person to think of something else which grows into a larger, more exciting, but not always pleasant story as we go along. That's what happened one afternoon as another aide and I helped a curmudgeon named Sam. He couldn't see or hear well so he became cranky very quickly when he was confused about what was going on around him. He raised his voice and shouted at us.

As we transferred Sam into his wheelchair to take him to the evening meal, he ordered, "Bring my pickup around front so I can leave soon."

"Your pickup isn't here," I said much too quickly.

Before I could add that his daughter had it, Sam yelled at me excitedly, "Someone stole my pickup!"

"No, --- ," I began.

Interrupting me, Sam shouted, "Call the law now and report this!"

The nurse came to my rescue. "I already did."

"What did they say?" Sam asked.

67

"That they'd get right on it and let you know in the morning. Things like this take time you know," she explained.

"I suppose it does," he conceded softly.

Another day I was helping Sam with his bath. Baths are a chore that people with Alzheimer's fear. I found that Sam, as well as some of the other residents dispositions, stayed more mellow during the dreaded bath if I could keep up a running conversation.

So I started with, "That was some rain we had last night. I saw on the news that the river was out of its banks in Cedar Rapids and flooded some streets."

"Where at?" Sam perked up with interest.

"It was at Ellis Park and over Edgewood Road I think."

"Oh no, my boat probably washed away. I wish you had told me sooner so I could have drug the boat up in the yard by my house," he groaned.

"Oh, you live there?" Great! Of all things to tell him, I had to mention a flood around his house.

Sam answered, "I've lived there for years. My house is up on the hill above the boat dock. I keep my boat tied at the dock in the summer and carry it up in my yard by the house in the winter. Now I've lost my boat," he groaned.

"No, you didn't, Sam." I tried to make amends. "I heard the water was rising so I had your boat carried up into the yard for you. It's safe and sound now."

Rescuing his boat was the least I could do after I had worried the poor fellow so much. At least by then before I could say anything else to upset Sam, his bath was over.

I hadn't done my homework on Sam. It seemed I kept bringing up the wrong subjects with him. I needed to make a list of things not to talk about to him. Let's see --- his pickup, his boat, and floods at Ellis Park for starters.

20.

It's All In The Eyes Of The Beholder

It's been awhile since I've played with dolls, and I don't ever remember having an imaginary friend, but in recent years I have known people who did. For someone with dementia, the reality of the moment might not always be the same for them as it is for the rest of us. The quicker we learn to accept that fact and play along, the easier it will be for people with Alzheimer's to exist in our world.

One afternoon at the care center, I sat down at the table with a frail, petite lady named Lora to feed her a candy bar she won at bingo.

I noticed she seemed fidgety. "What's the matter, Lora?"

"I have had company all afternoon, and he won't leave," she said irritated.

"Who was it?" I looked around and saw no one.

"I don't know who he is, but he's ten years old."

"Where is he now?"

"He's sitting on the wheel of my chair," she said in a hushed voice as she looked sideways without moving her head.

The message was finally sinking in. I had thought the children from elementary school next door had been visiting before I came to work, but now I knew differently. The wheels on Lora's chair were much too narrow and close to the side of her wheelchair for anyone to sit on, besides there wasn't anyone there.

"He isn't here now. He must have left," I said to calm her down.

"Oh, you think he's gone?" Lora asked.

"Yes, he must have gone home."

"His mother probably came home from work and called him," Lora decided, relaxing now that we were alone.

"Probably," I agreed.

One Sunday afternoon a few weeks later at snack time, I sat down by Lora at the table to help her with a piece of coconut pie.

"Boy, this is good! Have you got another piece of this pie?" She asked.

"You want another piece?" I was surprised since Lora was not a very big eater.

"No, not for me. For my friend."

"Where is your company now?" Seeing no one, I thought her visitor may have left.

"He's right here in this chair beside me," Lora confided, nodding her head sideways at the empty chair.

I caught on quicker that time. "Okay, let me help you with your pie first then I'll go back and get him a piece."

Lora turned to the empty chair, and said in a grandmotherly tone, "You wait until she gets done helping me then she'll get you some pie, too."

Hearing the tone brought me to ask, "How old is your friend?"

"He's ten years old."

"What's his name?" I asked, realizing this must be the same *friend* that visit Lora a few weeks before.

"He's never told me," Lora sounded baffled by that.

After I finished feeding her the pie, I asked, "Now do you still want me to get your friend a piece of pie?"

Glancing at the empty chair and then back at me, Lora said in disdain, "No, not now. Can't you see that he just left?"

Not missing a beat, I replied, "Of course, I can now. How did I miss that."

Lora had the same imaginary friend return frequently to visit her, and more often than not, she enjoyed his company. Perhaps it kept her from being lonely for a time, and that's what friends are for, isn't it? Next time I'm there when he comes to visit I won't mind entering Lora's reality to talk to the little boy if I can, because that's what I did you know. I entered her reality. Why I'd be glad to get him a piece of pie. Sometime, I might even ask him to tell Lora and me his name.

21.

Orange Sunflower Hot Pads

Jenny, an outspoken lady who liked to stay busy, spent much of her time crocheting potholders from donated yarn. As soon as she finished one, she'd give it away to the aides then start another one.

One morning, I looked into her room. My attention was caught by a large, hot pad the size of a dinner place on Jennie's lap. It was a different pattern than the square pot holders she had made before. It consisted of two sunflowers with a brown background holding them together to make it thick enough to set hot pans on. I had recently painted my kitchen walls bright yellow and put up a border that hugged the ceiling: yellow sunflowers against a dark green background.

Looking at that sunflower hot pad made me wonder if she could make two like that for me to hang on my kitchen wall. Although I crochet, I thought this task would be something to keep Jenny busy. Everyone needs something to do. They should have a purpose in life even if they live in a care center.

So I ventured in the room and asked, "That sunflower

hot pad matches my kitchen border, Jenny. If I brought in some yarn, could you make me two of those?"

"I guess so," she said slowly as though she had to think about it, but all too quickly, I took her answer as a yes.

The next day, I brought yellow, brown and dark green skeins of yarn to work with me and left them with Jenny. I gave her instructions to make the middle of the flower brown. The petals should be yellow and the background dark green to match my border.

A few days later, Jenny called me into her room to get my approval of her work so far. She held up the sunflower she'd crocheted which had a light green middle and orange petals. That was not the yarn that I gave Jenny.

"Oh, I thought the flower was going to have a brown middle with yellow petals, Jenny."

"I thought you'd like these colors better. I think it's pretty."

"Oh yes, it is," I began, trying to figure out how to keep from hurting her feelings. "The thing is the sunflowers in the border on my kitchen wall have brown middles and yellow petals. I wanted to hang the hot pads on the wall so I wanted them to match the border. Do you still have the yarn I gave you?" I was afraid Jenny may have already made someone else a square potholder out of my yarn

Jenny pointed beside her chair. "Yes, it's right down there."

"Could you please make the sunflowers those colors for me?"

"Okay," she said reluctantly, because she knew she'd have to go to the trouble of tearing out the work she had already done.

A few days later, Jenny called me back in to see the sunflowers. The middle was brown and the petals were yellow, but now the trim around the petals was brown, too.

"These are nice, Jenny, but ....," I paused, beginning to feel guilty for complaining. "I need the row on the outside to be dark green. Do you still have the skein of dark green yarn I gave you?"

"Yes, but I thought you might want the outside to match the middle of the sunflower." Jenny looked at me as though she couldn't believe how picky I was.

By now, I had decided that I'd have been better off if I had crocheted the hot pads myself. "It's just that the dark green matches the border on my walls. I'm sorry about this," I apologized.

"That's all right. I'll fix them for you." Jenny spoke in a calm, deliberate voice, trying her best to be patient with me.

A few more days passed before Jenny again called me into her room. I was expecting to see a completed hot pad. What she handed me was two separate sunflowers, the petals trimmed in dark green like I wanted, but thin and curling up, because they weren't crocheted together.

"I have these two done now." Jenny sounded relieved that the difficult task was over.

"I see that, but are you going to hook them together to make one hot pad?"

Jenny's relief turned to one of disbelief that I still wanted more. "I thought these were pretty just like they are!"

"Of course, they are, but they'd be thicker if they were crocheted together." I hated to ask once more if she had all the yarn I had given her which should have made three or four sunflower hot pads. "Where is the hot pad you went by for a pattern. Maybe we could look at it again." I thought Jenny may have forgotten how to put the hot pad together.

"Well, I gave it back," she admitted.

"It wasn't yours?"

"No, it belonged to someone else. I just borrowed it. It looked too hard for me to put together so I gave it back. These sunflowers look okay like they are, don't they?"

When I saw the hopeful look on Jenny's face I had no other choice. "Sure they do! They'll look great hanging on my kitchen wall." I assured her.

It was time to give up. This was as good as those sunflowers were going to get. Without the original hot pad to look at, I couldn't put them together either.

A few days later, Jenny called me into her room. Laying on her lap was a completed sunflower hot pad which the gleeful lady held up for me to see. "Look what I have."

"Did you make that one?" I was thinking her crocheting had really improved. It sure looked better than the two curly petal sunflowers she crocheted for me.

"No, the lady down the hall gave it back to me. She said she had no use for it, and maybe I could use it for a pattern." Jenny held it out to me, smiling. "The ones I made for you were too hard to make so I'll never make another one. You take this one home and use it. She'll never know the difference."

Now hanging on my kitchen wall, I have the original sunflower hot pad, two I made (in the colors I wanted) and right along side them hang Jenny's two curly petal sunflowers just like I promised her. I'm glad after all I put Jenny through to crochet what she must have thought was my very particular order that she managed to get those sunflowers made for me. I could have finished the sunflowers into one hot pad now that I had the original to go by, but I didn't. I look at those curly sunflowers and smile as I remember the lesson that Jenny's patience taught me.

Something like crocheting that Jenny had done all her life and had once seemed so easy for her to do had became a struggle. I appreciated how hard she tried to please me, and the frustration she felt at not being able to understand how to get the hot pad to look just like the original pad.   It brought back to me the struggles my father had with tasks that had once been simple. I saw his frustration at not being able to complete those tasks, and how he felt when he didn't understand why he couldn't. Looking through that window in my memory makes me wonder if I could be in Jenny's and my father's situation some day. If that day comes, I pray that my caregivers have the patience to let me do as much as I can even if the task is not completed to perfection. I hope that they will care enough to understand the confusion I'm going through at that time in my life and praise the effort I made even if the project isn't done to their satisfaction.

22.

You're Always Wrong

Being wrong is something we learn to deal with when we take care of people with AD. The customer is always right, and we are always wrong. The person who has Alzheimer's is living in his or her own reality, and they think they are always right.

One day, Norma called an aide into her room to look for a bug she said crawled under her bed. The aide got down on her hands and knees, peered under the bed, and couldn't find the bug so she left.

Several times that evening, Norma put on her call light, and whoever answered, at Norma's insistence, had to get down on their hands and knees to look under her bed. No one could find the bug, but Norma was sure she saw it go under there. She refused to go to bed for fear the bug would crawl up the covers and get in bed with her. When we had no luck finding the bug, she turned on the call light again and again.

"What kind of bug was it?" The aide asked as she got down to peer under the bed for the umpteenth time.

"A Mexican beetle," Norma declared.

The aide slowly lifted her head from the floor to view the serious look on Norma's face.

Changes of finding a Mexican beetle under that bed was slimmer than winning the lottery so the aide didn't want to keep getting down on her hands and knees all night. The aide lowered her head to the floor again.

"Oh, there he is!" She said as she made a swipe under the bed, then sat back up with a clinched hand. "I got that bug. I'll throw him away now." She stood up, walked over to the wastecan, opened her hand and deposited the "Mexican beetle".

"Are you sure that was the right bug?" Norma wasn't convinced.

"Oh, yes. I'm sure," the aide assured her.

"Really are you sure? How can you tell?" Norma quizzed her.

The aide knew Norma wasn't going to give up easily now that she had worried for hours about that bug. Most likely in a few minutes, she would have her light on again to declare that the bug she saw was still under her bed.

Looking down in the waste can again, the aide replied, "I know I killed the right bug. It's a Mexican beetle all right."

"Yes, but how do you know it is?" Norma asked unrelenting.

"I can see his sombrero," the aide confirmed.

With that for proof that the bug would no longer bother her, Norma relaxed and went to bed. She just needed to know that she had been right about seeing that bug. Right down to it's nationality and how it was dressed.

Paranoia and hallucinations are symptoms that happen to people with Alzheimer's. Strange thoughts and sights can cause a person and their caregiver many anxious moments. It's so natural for the caregiver to want to say the person with Alzheimer's is wrong about what they think or see. Trying to explain the truth only angers a person who is so sure he/she is right. Whether it be a resident in a care center or a person in his/her own home, We need to be prepared by learning how to defuse their anxious moments, because once those symptoms rear their ugly heads, a long, discomforting journey has just begun.

I went through one such horrible journey with my parents. After over half century of being happily married, my father decided my mother was seeing another man. He felt that she intended to leave him. A painful accusation that was hard for my mother, who was so very hurt by it, to live through. What she didn't realize was that almost always someone with Alzheimer's disease will suspect the person closest to them of trying to harm them in someway. Those thoughts might not last long or they may last for months. Always through the long ten years of hell we lived in while Dad was ill, my mother had trouble coping with how my father reacted to the different symptoms of Alzheimer's, but she endured. For that I am thankful and so was my father, because he died peacefully with her at his side.

When Dad's paranoid thoughts about Mom leaving began to wane, and we thought the worst was over along came hallucinations which was more exaggerated by the fact that he had sundowning. Dad tended to wander through the house during the night, get lost and wind up sleeping in a chair or another bed, because he couldn't find his bedroom once he left it. So one morning, I showed up at my parents home to help out. Dad was sitting in a chair, wedged between the microwave oven stand and the refrigerator. He looked tired, nervous and very upset.

Getting both of us some coffee, I placed the cups on the table and invited Dad to come join me. He sat down. I asked him what was wrong, and he began his tale. Now my dad had always been a wonderful story teller. Everyone loved to listen to him tell about his early days of horses, model T's, picking fruit and cotton out west and hard days struggling to make ends meet during the depression. This tale was much different from those.

Dad said he got up in the night to go to the bathroom and heard whistles coming from outside. He looked out a bedroom window and saw men running from tree to tree in the front yard. They seemed to be trying to figure out how to best rush the house and get in to steal his car keys. For the moment, Dad had forgotten that he hadn't seen his car keys for sometime. We hid them.

In those days seeing things that weren't there was a new concept to me. Immediately, I suggested that Dad must have been dreaming. His face reddened and he yelled at me, "I don't lie. If I say I saw men in the yard, I did."

Surprised by the outburst which was so uncharacteristic of him, I knew I had to suggest something different. It came to me then not to try and change what Dad was thinking because he was so sure he was right. Just defuse the situation by getting him on another subject. So I told him that those men were gone when I drove in. So he didn't need to worry. They had given up and left. That settled Dad down except for the fact that he threatened to shoot anyone who tried to force their way into his home.

That presented a whole new problem. Dad had always been a hunter and had several guns on a rack at the foot of the bed. What if some night, he saw Mom move in bed and imagined she was an intruder. He might shoot her. For Mom's safety, I felt I had no choice but to take his guns home with me when he wasn't looking. Of course, I felt like a thief stealing his guns, and laid a guilt trip on myself which took me some time to work through.

Another example of caregivers being less than perfect in the eyes of the care receiver is in this story about Sam, the curmudgeon. He woke up on the wrong side of the bed most of the time. It seemed the aides could never do anything right when dressing him or transferring him to his wheelchair. Since he couldn't see or hear well, he was always worried about what was happening to him. It was understandable that he would be fearful.

One day, Sam's daughter came to visit. I warned her that Sam seemed extra cranky that day.

"Dad, have you been out of sorts today? What are you acting like that for?"

"Who said I was out of sorts?" He shouted at her.

"One of the girls that takes care of you said so," the daughter told him.

"Oh, that," he muttered, then not realizing that I was in the room, he confided in his daughter, "Well, I have to act like that to them so they don't run over me. I have to let them know who's boss."

"You have to be nice to the girls. They are only trying to help you, Dad," the daughter scolded.

Now I understood Sam. Elderly people lose most of their independence when they become ill and enter the care center. Since he couldn't see or hear well, he wanted to make sure he still had the upper hand so we would know that he was still in control.

One evening, I was pulling a full laundry barrel by Sam. I accidentally bumped his wheelchair.

Unable to make out more than blurred images, he shouted, "What the hell was that?"

Knowing that he was afraid because he couldn't see me or the barrel, I stopped to explain to him. "I'm sorry, Sam. I bumped your wheelchair with my laundry barrel. I didn't mean to do that. Are you all right?"

"I'll never live over it," Sam said dryly.

Of course, he was exaggerating, but Sam was still trying to grasp that upper hand by making me feel guilty. Then things changed one night at the evening meal.

I was helping Sam with his meal. He didn't like to be fed so if we put food on the spoon and handed it to him, he would feed himself. That night he hadn't eaten very much before he stopped. I tried to persuade him to eat more.

"I wish people would stop pestering me about eating," Sam yelled at me.

"But, Sam," I said calmly, "you didn't eat enough to keep a flea alive."

"I wish you would quit bothering me," he shouted. "I just don't eat very much."

"Neither does a flea," I said back to him.

Sam's face grew thoughtful as he tried to think of a retort, then he said quietly as he grinned at me, "You got me there."

All right! I'm not sure why, but chalk one up for me. At least, I made Sam grin.

23.

Translations Are Required

People with Alzheimer's disease call objects by the wrong name, or their minds go blank in the middle of a sentence. More frequently than not, they can't remember what they were going to say. Sometimes, they begin to use a language of their own making, or don't speak at all. Other times, they seemed to comprehend what is said to them, but sometimes when we don't understand what they try to say to us, they become frustrated and angry. We try to learn to translate by filling in the blanks, not correcting them when they use the wrong words and try to figure out what they're trying to tell us when they speak their own language.

John, a tall, thin man, had Alzheimer's disease and suffered from a stroke. He spoke clearly, but often used the wrong words.

He had a good sense of humor and would laugh often, but he did get frustrated easily and would strike out. We tried to do our best to interpret what he wanted so we could keep him from getting angry.

Always restless, John continually had his feet off the

steps of his wheelchair. One day, an aide bent over to put his feet back on the steps, and to him it was too tempting an opportunity. He slapped her on the bottom.

The aide straightened up fast, and looked to see why he was annoyed at her. "What did you do that for, John?"

John chuckled.

"Look at him. He was teasing you," I said.

"You be nice to me," the aide teased back. "I'm a nice girl."

John looked at her then said slowly, "You're more thanksgiving than I would have been."

John had meant forgiving instead of thanksgiving. If the situation had been reversed, he was trying to tell the aide he wouldn't have found his actions funny. I did find the story funny so I told it to his wife the next evening when she came to visit. Quietly, John sat listening to my every word.

In a few minutes, an aide came over, bent down to put John's feet on his steps, and his hand came up to hit her on the bottom. His wife stopped him this time. "Don't do that. You be nice to her. Did you see him?" She asked me. "He was going to do it again."

"He's just teasing," I told her, not wanting her to think we were upset with John.

"Well, he never did that to me at home," she said, grinning at her husband.

I could see John's wife was looking at his actions in an entirely different light than I had. "We'll keep reminding him of that," I said and laughed.

Unlike the way I accidentally brought up things that upset Sam, I discovered things about John that he liked to talk about.

Not long after John moved into the care center, another aide and I were helping him get ready for bed. John pointed behind us and said proudly, "He's a big sucker!"

We turned to see a wooden plaque on the wall with a trophy size, large mouth bass attached to it. I knew that John must have been an avid fisherman to have his prize catch mounted. We found when we wanted to get a chuckle out of him all we had to do was mention fishing.

Motion detector fish had just arrived on the market so I bought one. I took it to work to show John and some of the other residents. John loved that talking fish. His eyes lit up when he saw it, because it reminded him of his fishing days. I assured him that this rubber fish wasn't the prize catch that his bass was. At hearing that statement, John beamed proudly.

"Push the red button under the fish's stomach," I told him.

John stuck his long, crooked finger on the button and pushed. The fish swung its head around to face John and asked, "Are you looking at me?"

John's eyes grew large in surprise. A grin spread slowly over his face.

"What did that fish say to you?" I asked.

John chuckled and repeated, "Are you looking at me?"

"That's right. Now push the button again and see what else he says."

The fish, facing John, burst into a mournful tune about getting hooked, reeled in and wanting to be taken back to the water as his tail kept beat with the music. John couldn't resist sticking his finger in the fish's mouth to see if it would bite him. That didn't happen, but that fish had enough actions and sayings to keep John spellbound and grinning for sometime.

One more window I opened by accident for John was his connection with the United States flag. I was reading poems to the residents one afternoon. While I read a short poem about flags, I noticed John stared at me, listening intently. I remembered in his line of work as a postmaster he ran a flag up the flag pole every day.

"Did you put the flag on the flag pole at work, John?"
"Yes!"
"Did you do it every day?"
"More days than not."

"Sometimes the flags would wear out, and you probably had to buy a new one, didn't you?"

"Yes, I got new ones," he said with enthusiasm.

I found out later from his wife that John not only flew the flag at work, but he was involved with the American Legion. During a military funeral, it was John's job to fold the flag in the proper way that had been draped on the casket and present it to the family. He ordered new flags for the Legion so there was always a supply on hand for funerals and for replacing worn out flags. In that intent look he gave me was the memories of all the flags he had handled, and how proud he had been to have the opportunity to show his respect for our nation's flag. I was glad I looked up from reading long enough to see that moment when a window opened for John.

People with Alzheimer's disease hear what we say to them and process it better than we know sometimes. I remember a few times when I said something that I didn't explain clearly and had to make amends.

"I want to brush your dentures. Will you give them to me?"

"No, I won't give them to you. These are my dentures!"

"Let me put your shoes on for you."

"No, you can't wear my shoes. They are mine."

"Come with me, Joe. We'll take a bath."

"Oh, are you taking a bath with me?"

24.

All Her Babies Were Named June

A tiny, humped shouldered lady, Irene could be sweet of nature or a rascal whose demeanor was more that of a small child than an elderly person. She adopted each of us as part of her family, calling us Sissy or Mama. No one came to visit her at the care center so we assumed she didn't have a family. She loved dolls, and named each of hers June. She treated them as if they were real babies. It was a mystery to us why she gave all of her babies the same name so one day I asked her about it. She told me that June was her sister's name. That was all she could tell me, because her memory consisted usually of what was happening to her at the moment.

One day, two women came to visit Irene. Before they left, I had a chance to talk to them. The older woman said she was Irene's sister, and she shared Irene's story with me.

Irene and at least three other sisters had been placed in an orphanage when they were very small. This sister was too young to remember those days, but she had recently tracked down the addresses of her birth family and wanted to meet the siblings still living. She had another sister living close by and

Irene.

I explained that I wondered about the mystery of Irene's babies all bearing the name June, and that Irene had told me it was her sister's name. Being too young at the time of separation, the lady told me she didn't have any memory of the orphanage or the older sister, but she knew there had been one named June. Irene would have been old enough to remember. She did know June had taken care of the smaller sisters until each of them had been adopted. In the past few years, June had passed away.

Now the mystery was solved. Though she didn't remember much about her younger days, Irene did remember the good care and love she received from her sister. She showed her appreciation and honored her sister's memory by naming each of her babies after June. We need to keep the example of how Irene felt about her sister's loving caregiving in mind when we are taking care of others. They may not remember the care we have given them from one day to the next, but down deep, I'm convinced they'll always appreciate it just like Irene did.

25.

Two Kernels Of Corn In A Hill

Someone should write a book of sayings that were used close to a century ago. Something as simple as a phrase that was used to greet someone can have meaning for an elderly person with dementia.

One evening, I was taking residents to the assisted dining room. Each time I wheeled someone in, John would look at me and laugh.

"You're sure in a good mood," I commented.

"We've been having a talk, and he liked something I said," came a male voice from the back of the room. It was a volunteer who was tightening the screws on the podium in the corner.

"What did you say to him?"

"I asked him how he was, and he said okay. I told him I was as good as two kernels in a hill. He liked that."

"What does that mean?"

The volunteer explained, "Well, back in the horse drawn corn planter days when the farmer was planting corn he'd have to get off to see if the planter was putting out the right number of kernels in the hill. If there were two kernels in a hill, he was doing great, and if there wasn't he had to adjust the planter. So when farmers greeted each other seventy years ago, they'd say they were as great as two kernels in a hill."

Something so simple to say had brightened up John's day by opening a window to when he was young. After that I'd greet John with "You're as great as two kernels in a hill." That always made him smile.

26.

A Support Group Of Two

I threw this story in because whether people suffer from Alzheimer's or some other devastating illness, they need to feel that someone is there to listen when they need to talk. Then when the ability to communicate leaves them, maybe just our being there is a comfort.

Someone in failing health can take a fast turn for the worse sometimes. Though Julia, a plump, cheerful woman, had trouble with her vision, she liked to go for walks and would bring back flowers to her room. Then suddenly everything went dark for Julia. It hit her hard. She wanted to give up doing anything for herself. As sure as she was that she couldn't manage dressing or feeding herself anymore, we were just as sure she could do these tasks once she got over the shock of not being able to see. The problem was how to get her to that point.

I came up with an idea one day. We had another lady, Alice, who as a young girl had learned how to cope with being sightless. She had married, raised a family and kept her own house with the help of her husband and children. Her attitude was that she could do anything so I wondered if some of her confidence would wear off on Julia.

Sitting down by Julia, I said, "We'd like to see you be able to do some of the things that you were doing before you couldn't see."

Julia lamented, "I can't do anything anymore for myself."

"You know Alice and her husband that sit at the table near you in the dining room. She hasn't been able to see for years, and she does many things for herself. Would you like to talk to her about how she figured out to get the food on her spoon or to put her dress on right?"

"I guess so." Julia was reluctant.

"Okay, let me go ask Alice if she would like to visit with you." I hurried down to Alice's room before Julia could change her mind.

"Hello, Alice. Could I talk to you a minute?"

"Sure, come on in."

"I wondered if you could help me out with something. You know Julia that sits near you in the dining room? She has completely lost her sight, and doesn't know how to help herself. We aren't sure what to do to help her make the decision to try to do things for herself. Since you have been taking care of yourself for a long time, I wondered if you could talk to her. You could give her some tips on how to do things such as how to feed herself or dress herself."

"Okay, if you think it would help, I'd be glad to do it," Alice said eager to help.

"Swell, could you do it right now if I took you to Julia's room?"

"Sure."

Back in Julia's room I introduced Alice to her. "Julia, I have brought you some company. Remember I told you I'd go see if Alice would like to talk to you? Well, she is here with me. I thought maybe you could ask her questions about how to do things, and what it has been like for her not to see all these years."

"Okay," Julia agreed slowly.

"Just push your call light when you two are done talking so I can take Alice back to her room."

As I left, Alice was saying that she had been blind for almost seventy years so she knew what she was talking about. Later, when the call light came on, I went back to get Alice. On the way down the hall, I asked her how she thought the meeting had gone. Had Julia seemed interested in what she was saying? Perhaps it would take more than one meeting for Alice's enthusiasm to catch hold of Julia. Not only could Alice describe ways to help Julia to do things in their dark world, but they could talk about feelings they shared in common that we could only guess at. At least, Alice cared enough to try to help Julia.

27.

Which Side Is Mine

Sometimes to make it easier to take care of a resident, the furniture in their side of a double room is changed around. With so many sudden changes in their lives and minds, they have trouble adjusting to the room they now live in. Add to that the fact that the beds and closets are switched to the opposite side of the room and that makes for real confusion. One thing that someone with Alzheimer's disease doesn't like is any sort of change in routine or location.

When I came to work, I heard the story of 95 year old Charlie's efforts to move his roommate's heavy clothes closet across to what had been Charlie's side of the room after housekeeping had made a switch in furniture. When asked what he was doing, he replied that this was the closet that had his clothes in it. He wanted it back on his side of the room. The aides explained to him that the closet Charlie was pushing wasn't his. The closet on what was now his side of the room had Charlie's clothes in it. They pushed the roommate's closet back to where it had been, and left. They thought Charlie was confused since they didn't see an underlying cause for him wanting to move the closet.

When I went to get Charlie for his bath, I happened to look on the wall back of his bed and saw his roommate's wooden name plaque. Above the head of Charlie's bed was a framed crocheted name doily belonging to the roommate, plus there were other mementos of the roommate's on the wall as well.

On the roommate's side of the room, Charlie's large collage of family pictures still hung. More family pictures were on the wall over the roommate's bed.

In somewhat of a hurry, the furniture, which all looks identical, had been switched in the room, but the personal items on the wall that in his mind identified that side of the room as Charlie's hadn't been moved. No wonder he was confused about where he belonged and what belonged to him. I would have been, too.

Maybe sometimes we are too quick to label people with dementia, who act out of the ordinary, as being confused. We should slow down and look at the situation to see if there's something they have been trying to tell us all along.

28.

A Caregiver's Sense Of Humor

Whether you are a caregiver in a home or a care center, having a good sense of humor makes the days go by easier. When we are able to laugh, it lifts our spirits, and as caregivers, we see much that touches us deeply so we need to learn how to smile and laugh more to keep our spirits up. Our good natured caregiving in the nursing home is depended upon by the people we take care of who have moments of sadness and depression when they think about what has happened to them. Hopefully, our laughter will be the infection of the day that we wouldn't mind seeing spread through the facility. In fact, we have learned that our moods, whether it be a happy one, angry or sad, are mirrored by people who have dementia.

Janie, a tall, slim lady, could be cheerful and easy going, but other times, she could be cross and suspicious of the aides every move.

Luckily, I caught up with her on what was a good day for her to tell her it was time to take a shower.

"I thought of that early this morning when I saw the line outside the bathroom door, but I got busy doing something else and forgot about the shower," Janie explained to excuse her memory lapse.

"Oh, that's okay. I don't mind reminding you when it's time to take your shower," I told her.

"Well, I hope you remember to tell me before I get moldy."

I looked at her a moment wondering how to answer her, then she smiled and repeated, "I don't want to go long enough that I get moldy."

"Oh, of course not. We'd never let you go that long before you had a bath," I replied, laughing at the thought of a green Janie.

Worried that I might forget to come get her for a bath, Janie seemed to be hinting that I might be as forgetful as she was. That left me I wondering what she'd heard.

As I've mentioned before my father, for most of his life, was a wonderful story teller who elaborated on stories about his youthful experiences with a sense of humor that kept everyone listening and laughing. When Alzheimer's destroyed that part of his brain, he forgot the stories he used to tell, but he could still come back with a one liner now and then to get a laugh.

One day at the doctor's office, the nurse came into the exam room. She said hello to my mother and me then turned to my dad, "How are you today, Bill?"

"I must be okay. I'm not dead yet," he said, smiling.

"Oh, Bill, you're okay. You still have your sense of humor," the nurse teased.

"I'm glad of that. It's the only sense I have left now," Bill said.

"Well, Bill," the nurse shot back at him, "if I had to lose all my senses but one I'd want to be able to keep my sense of humor just like you have."

From the smile on his face, I'd say that's just what Dad

needed to hear.

The old saying that you are as young as you feel must be true. At least a gentleman named Lester, a tall, man who smiled easily and had a great sense of humor, believed it. Longevity ran in his family so at 102 years of age, Lester was still walking in the care center halls with the assist of a walker and the accompaniment of an aide.

Early one morning on the way to breakfast, Lester walked briskly up the hall, but he wasn't too sure the much younger woman walking beside him was an energetic as he was. That 102 year old man turned to the aide, smiling from ear to ear. "What's the matter? Am I walking too fast for you?"

As long as the caregiver is laughing with the person and not at him/her, that's the best medicine we have at the moment with no cure for this devastating disease on the horizon yet.

Laughter is the closest distance between two people --
Victor Borge

29.

The Scrapbook

The stories on these pages are mostly recollections of events I have seen at the care center. Through my experiences, I've learned it was much harder to open a window for someone we don't know anything about than it had been for me with my father. That's why I like to talk to family members to get to know the residents better.

I like to feel I opened windows for my father all the time since I was so close to him. He was content in his home most of the time except for the usual Alzheimer's symptoms when he thought he heard robbers trying to break into the house. Or when his mind started it's reverse trip to his youth, he'd get restless and want to go home to the house he lived in as a younger, healthy man in Vernon County, Missouri, raising a family on his 80 acre farm.

Dad liked exploring the five acres he owned near Keystone, Iowa. He had the run of the place with my mother and me keeping an eye on him. Because I shared my dad's love of the outdoors, I'd keep him company on his park bench in the back yard quite often. We'd watch the birds flit about, and we'd wave at the neighbors who honked as they drove by. Sometimes we'd sit quietly, watching his garden grow. Once in a while, I'd seize the opportunity to cut and clean Dad's fingernails which Mom seemed to neglect, because Dad wasn't keen on her messing with his nails. Sitting in that peaceful, fresh air, Dad was more receptive to letting me fuss over him.

There was one time I remember opening a window that sent Dad's memory back into his childhood.

Mom had been doing spring cleaning upstairs when she found on a closet shelf a very old scrapbook. Long in length and narrow in width, the book cover had painted on it a knight and maiden staring lovingly at each other. The maiden's bright green dress took up most of the picture. The knight wore a red outfit with white tights and atop his head was a red, Robin Hood hat. A brass bracket with a keyhole in it was attached to the cover, but the latch was missing. So was the key. Its pages were brittle and fragile, yellowed with age. Each page was solid with a paper covering over it containing two gold trimmed holes for the pictures to be inserted between.

Mom asked me if I knew where the book came from. I didn't so I suggested that she ask my two brothers if they remembered it.

By that time, Dad had been outside for a while. It was time to check to see if he was still on the park bench and talk him in to coming back into the house. So I went outside to bring him in, seated him at the table and got us each a cup of coffee. The invitation to sit with me at the kitchen table with coffee always was enough to get Dad indoors.

I pushed the scrapbook over in front of him and not expecting an answer, I asked, "Do you know where this scrapbook came from?"

"Sure, it belonged to my dad," he answered without any hesitation.

"It did?" I'd never dreamed it had such a long ago history. My grandfather died in 1924 when my father was twelve years old.

"Yes, he never liked us kids to play with it so when he left the house I'd sneak it down off the shelf and play with it, because I knew I wasn't supposed to have it."

"How did we get it?"

"Your brother, John, found it in the junk pile behind my mother's house when she moved to Nevada. Whoever helped her pack had thrown it away, because the lock was broken." He smiled fondly at the memory of how sneaky he had been as a child to play with that scrapbook when his father left the house.

In amazement, I marveled at how well my father's memory was working at the moment because he had that old scrapbook in front of him.

Later, I took snapshots of Dad's parents large, wedding picture that hung above Mom and Dad's bed. One day, I gently slipped one of my pictures into the first brittle page of the scrapbook and placed the closed book in front of my father. He opened it up and saw his parents picture. While he gave them a long, loving look, I snapped his picture. I had not only opened a window for my father, but I had a picture of Dad to remember the moment by, with his facial expressions looking more like the father I knew before Alzheimer's became a part of his life.

30.

The Floating Feathers of Yesterdays

If only the words I chose to comfort her with would have made a difference, but I realized, after so much time had passed, the well chosen words that once may have helped couldn't comfort her anymore. I looked at that frail, sweet lady who should have been filled with a century of wonderful memories and wisdom and knew that each day more was stolen from her as Alzheimer's disease covered her brain.

If you could have named a hymn or Christmas carol, she could still sing it. If you could have listened to me read to her, you'd have seen her pretty smile spread upward to light her dim eyes. If you could have eavesdropped on her while she carried a cheerful conversation between herself and her late husband, you'd have heard her let out a hearty chuckle. On the surface of her soul remained the emotional ability to laugh or cry depending on the moment.

A tall, much too thin lady who spoke in a coarse voice with a subdued demeanor, her memories were fleeting wisps that floated through her mind like fluffy down. Thoughts all too quickly gone before she had a chance to hold onto them long enough to speak them.

I'll forever be grateful for that special moment which was only to come by once. I happened to be sitting beside this woman, talking to her. I didn't expect a response, but she looked up at me. Something about the look on her face seemed more like her old self when she offered me a piece of profound advice that over time had been hidden away in her brain in a cover of plaque. "When you have lived as long as I have, first you will lose your knowledge then you'll lose your confidence."

Thinking that was all she had to say on the subject, I was about to leave when this woman, who rarely carried a conversation, spoke again. "I have a story about a little boy who lost yesterday. Want to hear it?"

"I'd like to hear your story," I encouraged.

She began in a sad, sing song fashion, "There once was a little boy who discovered that he had lost yesterday. He was very sad about that. The little boy hunted everywhere, but he couldn't find yesterday so he decided to ask his mother to help him.

"Mother," he said "I've lost yesterday, and I can't find it. Can you help me look for it?"

His mother could tell her little boy was very upset, and she wanted to comfort him so she said, "Son, you know there isn't much you can do when you lose yesterday. It's gone forever if you can't find it. You have today, and hopefully, you'll have tomorrow. You'll have to make due with that."

The little boy still felt bad about losing yesterday, but he decided his mother was right, and he was glad he had asked her to help him understand."

Suddenly, the lady stopped talking as the feather of memory floated on out of her grasp. Passively, she looked down at her hands folded in her lap which is the way I usually saw her. At first, I was speechless that so many words strung together in a story came from this woman who for a very long time hasn't had much to say. Then I complemented her on

103

telling me that very good story and thanked her for sharing it with me. Words that went over her as though I had never spoken them.

If only the words I spoke had some comfort for her, but I realized looking at that sad face whatever I said would float away like the feather. Reaching over, I patted her hands so she knew that I was with her. Hopefully, she might feel some reassurance from my presence and touch. To say to her everything would be all right wasn't going to help, because she had to feel down deep in her soul what I already knew. Things wouldn't be all right for her ever again. In her simple story about the little boy, she defined for me one of the ways Alzheimer's disease had affected her. It was her way of letting me know that it was her the disease had robbed of yesterdays.

This story won first place in an Iowa Health Care Association contest, but that isn't what makes this particular story special to me. What makes it special is the fact that I spent time with a group of people who had Alzheimer's. I let them talk about their memories, with some prompting of course.

The wise woman in the story had always been able to share her wisdom with everyone, but suddenly found she couldn't grasp anything in her memory to share with the group. Out of desperation, she tried to explain why she couldn't remember. This was the story she told me. I wrote it down, knowing that she was telling me to the best of her ability what many other people with AD want to say and can't.

I've always felt blessed that I took the time to listen to what this woman said and really understand what she tried to tell me. I began to think about how much we as caregivers are missing from other people's wisdom just like my wise lady by not taking the time to spark a memory or hear their stories. Even if we hear a story, do we really listen? Do we remember the details? Take it from me, the day will come when many of you will say you wished you'd asked questions about your family's past. We need to do that before Alzheimer's disease robs our loved ones minds of their memories. Taking notes or recording a story are easy ways to get the facts preserved for our memories.

31.

Super Aide

How often do we get asked what we do for a living? How often do you caregivers say you're just a housewife, you just take care of your wife, or in my case just a CNA? We have got to remember what we do is very important. I have been both a homemaker and a CNA. They are both very important jobs and so is caregiving. Don't sell yourself short.

For caregivers in the home that find the thought of giving up a loved one to the care of a nursing home so very difficult, I can say I've been a caregiver in both worlds. There comes a time for the sake of the caregiver's own health that they have to give in to seeking help. Statistics tell us that 8 out of 10 caregivers die before the care receiver. The loved one winds up getting taken care of by others in spite of all the caregiver's loving efforts so give serious thought about the day that's inevitably going to come when you need help. It might mean the difference between you not being around anymore or being able to still comfort the person you love when he/she needs you.

I'll tell you something that makes sense to me that I heard not too long ago. When you as a caregiver find yourself hesitating at your front door, hating to go back inside then you know it's time to find help. You're stressed out, exhausted, and your health is at steak. That doesn't make for a good caregiver. Your loved one deserves the best care.

With that thought in mind, I wrote this essay with super aide being a combination of the very dedicated caregivers in long term care.

"Hello," the lady in white said cheerfully to the wheelchair bound welcoming committee that greeted anyone entering the care center's front door. She stopped by one frail lady, patted her small, arthritic hand and asked, "How are you today?"

The aide waited for a reply, hoping at the very least for a twinkle of recognition in the older lady's faded brown eyes as she peered over the rim of her glasses. The aide was rewarded with a sweet smile.

This heath care worker performs many caregiving tasks during the day. She helps to keep the residents minds active by bringing in the world outside of the care center through conversations about the weather, current events, and news about happenings in the community. Also, she keeps them interested in what is going on around them in the care center by inviting them to participate in the daily activities. By talking about the next meal, she has them looking forward to joining the other residents in the dining room.

Sometimes the caregiver helps set aside the loneliness that grabs the elderly people she cares for by looking at a greeting card with them or by admiring a gift they received in the mail. When their poor eyesight prevents them from reading printed words, she reads the residents letters from their loved ones or an article in the newspaper. She listens to their stories from the past and about concerns that they face today, because they need someone to talk to, and this caregiver is there. She helps residents enjoy the moments when their moods are happy ones, and works to cheer them up when they are sad.

She tries to make the holidays a happy event for the residents instead of sad memories or lonely times. She hopes that each and every one of the people under her care are remembered by loved ones; not only with gifts but by sharing their time with the residents.

The aide's concern shows as she keeps a vigil over the residents that aren't feeling well. All the while, she tries to think of innovative ways to get them to eat and drink more liquids. She praises the residents courage for enduring to completion the tasks that are difficult for them, and she efficiently assists them with activity of daily living skills that they need help to perform.

She appreciates the residents willingness to confide in her and the fact that they worry about her traveling to and from the care center in bad weather. She finds it very touching when they say they'll miss her on her days off.

Her touch is gentle as she holds a limp hand, sharing her strength as she tries to let that person know that she is there. Her eyes mist over and a tear trickles down her cheek as she says a final good bye before she goes onto her other duties.

This is a cheerful, patient, understanding caregiver whose caring ways touches others. Does she sound like Super Aide to you? Think about it. What she does is not that hard to do. She is giving of herself unselfishly to care for others, and the fond gratitude she gets in return from those appreciative people is her reward.

People with goals succeed because they know where they're going. -- Earl Nightingale

32.

Caring About Coworkers And Yourself

Everyone knows a shift at the nursing home goes faster and the tasks are made easier if the aides all work together as a team, but we are all made differently as people. Sometimes it takes patience when we have to work with someone whose personality grates on our nerves, or we get exasperated when we feel that a fellow worker hid out when there was a task to do. Some aides work slower than others, and we have to learn to work around them as well as with them. The disturbing thought comes to our mind that we all get paid the same, and they should do their share of the work load.

Stop and give some thought to your coworkers. Does someone's personalty annoy you? We're all different as individuals, and there's not much we can do about that. We may need to count to ten (make that twenty), or whatever it takes to learn to work together in harmony in the work place.

People all work and play at their own pace. Some are faster than others from the time they are born. Not much can do to change that either unless a slow moving person learns to pick up speed on their own. The important and number one objective is that the aides do a good job, because the residents are depending on them.

It takes patience to help a new employee to learn the routine the way established aides are used to doing it. Most often, the new aide catches on fast, but there is always one that doesn't seem to figure out what needs to be done as fast as the other aides would like. Did you ever think that perhaps it is just a matter of giving that person a little more time? Most of us remember how nerve racking it was to start a new job. There was the nervous feeling of being under inspection, and when something went wrong that we were involved in, we'd feel lower than an ant. We need to make the new aides feel welcomed and give them a chance, because we caregivers are in danger of becoming a rare breed. We need to be protected by our employers and fellow employees before we become extinct. At the present time, there never seems to be enough of us to go around so give the new person on the job a chance. Then maybe before you know it, everyone will be working as a team.

The important thing to remember is that people need us to care for them. The priority is the people you are taking care. They deserve the best care from all of us as individuals as well as a team.

Every job is a self-portrait of the person who did it. Autograph your work with excellence. -- Unknown

33.

Job Burn out

Job burn out is prevalent. Stress sneaks up on everyone some time or other in their life, but stress doesn't come just from the job. It's very true that the health care worker's job is stressful with long, tiring shifts that causes emotions to run at bay. Sometimes we find it hard to face grieving the lost of a resident we became attached to.

The fact is that the caregiving job is only a portion of our day. The rest of the day we have our life outside of work to contend with. In this fast moving, complicated world we live in, we have all sorts of life's road blocks thrown at us. There are debts, broken marriages, single parenting, baby-sitter problems, sick children, unruly teenagers and the list goes on.

Can we help our fellow workers with what is wrong when they are stressed to the point that they carry their problem baggage with them to work? Probably not, but we can be sympathetic listeners and give them a little slack while they are going through the difficult time, working the problem out for themselves. It may not take long for a person to come to grips with a problem, and in the mean time, you still have a good worker on the job instead of one ready to quit. Just put yourself in that person's place. Next time it might be you with the problem so how would you want to be treated by your coworkers?

Learn to take care of yourself whether you are a health care worker or a caregiver at home. The caregiver at home happens to be tied to the situation for 24/7. Statistics show that 8 out of 10 caregivers died before the person they took care of. Stress plays a big part in a caregiver losing their health.

There will come a time when you, a caregiver, will need to seek help. The best time to do that is when you walk up to the front door of your house and don't want to enter. You have done the best job you can. Now it's time to get help.

Life shouldn't be all upsets and work. Find something that you like to do for fun like take a walk, paint a picture or sit down in a peaceful place to rest or read a book. Treat yourself to some relaxation.

It's hard to find the time, you say. Well, start right now. Take five minutes -- close your eyes, and picture that peaceful place in your mind. Breathe slowly in and out while you think pleasant thoughts about a favorite flower you like to smell, a fun place you'd like to visit or something funny you have heard.

Did you do it? Don't just stop with one time. This relaxation process is to be repeated as needed you know. That's my prescription to relieve stress. It's a start on the way to less stress so take it from there and be kind to yourself. It will not only help you to be a better person, but it will help you to be a better caregiver.

Now do you think that I have taken the time to practice all the above? No way, and I should have. For months, I'd been going full steam. I knew I was tired all the time. That didn't slow me down. I had too much to do. I think a couple friends from Colorado noticed I looked like I needed to slow down. They sent me a spa basket from Bath and Bed filled with a soft, fuzzy white robe, a candle, bath salts, a soft, soothing music CD, feet rubs, and lavender night lotion. I enjoyed the gift immensely, but it came too late. One morning, I had chest pains. My husband rushed me to the hospital ER, having a heart attack. After that warning signal have I slowed down? You bet I have. It's too bad I hadn't followed my own advice before it was too late.

"Happiness depends as nature shows, less on exterior things than most suppose." -- *William Cowper*

34.

Put Care In Caregiving

I worry about what will happen to me when I get old enough to need care. Just like everyone else, I hear and fear all the negative things. Maybe I'll never be placed in a care center, but again maybe I will be. It might not be one of my choosing so I worry about not being taken care of the way I would want to be.

Whether I get Alzheimer's disease or not, I have definite ideas about what kind of caregiving I want done for me. It's something that everyone should think about so you will be prepared for what's ahead in the not too distant future. As a caregiver, we should treat everyone we take care of like we'd like to be taken care of if the situation was reversed. (Sounds like the golden rule doesn't it?)

It's up to us as caregivers to work on making the home or care center we work in a better place for the people who live there. Make what is remaining of their lives as comfortable and fulfilling for them as you can with the thought that someday it might be you that needs care, and you'll expect the same quality of care in return.

The following is a list I've made that I intend to give to my caregivers when my time to need help arrives so they will be thoughtful about how they take care of me. The list was written to leave no doubt in their minds how I want to be taken care of.

1. I want you to look at me -- really look at me when I'm talking so you'll be able to understand what I am trying to tell you that I want. If I seem too slow to answer you back, I might not be able to process ideas well with my brain because of dementia. Give me a chance to speak when I'm ready.

2. Remember I have worked hard all my life, and now I have many aches and pains. Pay attention if I try to silently bear the pain. I might not be able to talk, or I might just be trying to keep from asking for help because I think I'm a bother. Be patient, look for silent signs that make you aware of my needs and help me.

3. Don't talk over my head about last night's party. Because I might not be able to hear well, you will confuse and scare me when you talk too fast. I won't comprehend what you are saying and be afraid you're talking about doing something to me that I won't like. That thought will scares me.

4. I expect I will be really, really old, and move slowly so don't try to make me move any faster, because I won't be able to walk as fast as you can. I might even consider a ride in a wheelchair a pleasure once in a while if you feel you have to get me to a meal or activity on your time schedule instead of mine.

5. Give me a drink of water often. My mouth gets so dry in this warm place, and I don't know how to get a drink for myself. I can't find it and am not even sure how to hold the glass up to my mouth so I need your help.

6. If someone wants to give me a sweet treat between meals, don't worry about that spoiling my supper, but stop to think how seldom I get a treat. Now that I have lost the taste for food something sweet tastes better to me than main meals.

7. If I want to eat my dessert before my meals, don't

stop me. At my age, I should be allowed to eat whatever I want to eat first, but pay close attention so you can figure out what my favorite foods are if I must eat some of everything on my plate. That's so you don't try to poke things in my mouth I don't like -- liver, beets, or green beans to start with. (I'm sure the list will be longer by the time I'm admitted.)

8. Feed me slowly so I have time to swallow. Don't put too big a bite in my mouth. My mouth isn't any bigger than yours except when you're yawning in my ear while I'm trying to eat.

9. After meals, wash the food off my mouth with a warm cloth, and for that matter, use a warm cloth in any other place you wash me. I won't like cold, wet wash cloths, and I don't think you would either.

10. Take me to the bathroom often. Sometimes I don't know when I need to go, and I can't find the bathroom by myself. I feel really embarrassed when I soil my pants. Don't make me feel bad.

11. Keep the path from my bed to the bathroom clear. I might try to get up to go by myself, and in the dim light with my poor eyesight, I might not see the strung out call light cord, walker, wheelchair, recliner, waste can, or bedside table. I may have forgotten something in that list that I would be sure to trip over so use your imagination. Or better yet take a moment to look around the room at the path I would take if I get up in the night. If you can't walk safely on that path with the lights on, then I sure can't in the dark.

12. Try to understand what I'm saying even though I don't speak like I should. Help me out if you can. The words are rattling around in my head, but it's hard for me to remember the right way to say them.

13. Be patient and kind when I feel frustrated and angry. I have many burdens to bear with the loss of my health, family, friends, and my home. Remember I can't be in a happy mood all the time. I suspect that you aren't either, and at your age, you have probably lost a lot less than I have at mine. Try

to understand.

14. I get colder than you do, because I sit still all the time, and my circulation is poor because my heart is bad. I shouldn't have to ask and might not think to so if I need a sweater, please go get it. If my feet get cold at night, please leave my socks on, just like I would have done at home, when you put me to bed and see to it that I have plenty of covers.

15. Move me once in a while when I've been up all day. My bottom is bony so it hurts me to sit in one position for a long time in an uncomfortable wheelchair.

16. Lay me down for a nap in the afternoon if I'm falling asleep in my chair. I need to rest, because I'm old and don't feel well. I don't like it when my head keeps nodding down and jerking up. It startles me, and makes my neck hurt.

17. Take off my shoes when I lie down for a nap. It doesn't save you much time later if you leave the shoes on, and it would sure make my hammer toes feel better to be free from those shoes. After all, I've probably worn them for the last ten years to walk in. I shouldn't have to wear them in bed, too.

18. Don't leave my lap robe, extra pillows or my shoes on top of my feet when you put me to bed. I'll sleep better if my feet aren't weighed down. They may be the only body part on me that I'm still able to move.

19. Don't rush around me when you help me with my activity of daily living skills without saying a word to me. Your silence bothers me. I can't decide if you are mad at me or don't like me. Please tell me what you are going to do next. I like to know what is ahead of me even if it's what you think of as a routine, simple thing such as putting on my nightgown, brushing what's left of my teeth, or taking that dreadful bath repeatedly.

20. Speaking of nightgowns, if I have any of my own, let me wear them even if you have to cut them up the back because I'm incontinent. If I am to consider this care center my home, then let me feel at home by sleeping in a pretty gown instead of a drab hospital gown. I may not feel the best, but

117

wearing those ugly gowns will make me feel even worse.

21. Don't just plop me in bed at night, wordlessly turn out the light and leave the room. It feels like the end for me. Take the time to say "Good night. I'll see you in the morning." even if you aren't the one who wakes me up. If those are the last words I hear at night maybe I'll drift off to sleep and dream about a new day ahead of me instead of fearing the worst is coming.

22. Leave a night light or table lamp on for me so I don't have to be in the dark. I won't be so frightened if I'm able to recognize that it's you coming in the room to check on me in the middle of the night. There's another important reason why I want a night light on. Maybe it's just my feelings on the subject but when my time comes to leave this world, I would rather not do it in the dark.

22. Above all take the time to smile at me when you're with me. That will help me feel safe. Once in a while, you could give me a hug, too. Don't be stingy with those, because if I'm able I'll give it right back to you.

Look for new releases coming soon by Fay Risner

Activities On A Shoestring Budget-For People With Late Stage Alzheimer's - Simple, cheap activities to do with people in mid to late state Alzheimer's.

Nonfiction at Fay's bookstore
http:www.booksbyfaystore.weebly.com

Hello Alzheimer's Good-bye Dad - about the author and her family's struggle to care for her father in his home.
Includes caregiver tips.

Floating Feathers Of Yesterdays – a three act play subject Alzheimer's

Other books include the Amazing Gracie Mystery Series
Neighbor Watchers book one
Specious Nephew book two
The County Seat Killer book three
The Chance Of A Sparrow book four
Moser Mansion's Ghosts book five

Ella Mayfield's Pawpaw Militia – Civil War Saga In Vernon County, Missouri

My Children Are More Precious Than Gold – Children – Historical fiction in Blue Ridge Mountains in Virginia

Two Amish Romance books
Christmas Traditions – Amish Love Story
A Promise Is A Promise – Nurse Hal Among The Amish Book One

The Dark Wind Howls Over Mary – western

Award Winning Short Story Collections
Butterfly And Angel Wings
A Teapot, Ghosts, Bats & More
Wild West Tales

Fay Risner's Bio

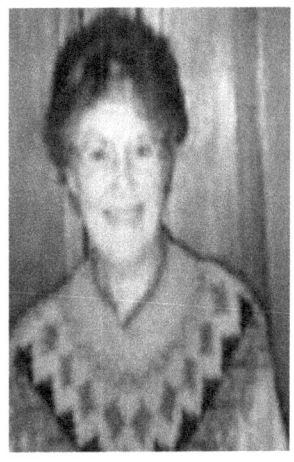

Fay lives with her husband, Harold, on a central Iowa acreage along with their sheep, milk goats, chickens, rabbits, cats and a dog. She is a retired Certified Nurse Aide and now divides her time between writing, and enjoying country life, gardening and fishing.

She has sold five stories to Good Old Days magazine and entered numerous story and essay contests. Fay has placed thirty four times. For more information about buying any of Fay's other books, about her life and interest plus her accomplishments and blog visit her website at http://www.booksbyfaybookstore.weebly.com

Accomplishments include Nurse Aide for 2004 awarded by the Iowa Health Care Association and 2006 Excellence for Professional Caregiver Award from Alzheimer's Association, Cedar Rapids, Iowa.

She is a volunteer on the Alzheimer's Association Outreach program since 1999 and until she retired facilitated a Alzheimer's support group in Keystone Nursing Care Center, Keystone, Iowa since 2000.

Notes

www.ingramcontent.com/pod-product-compliance
Lightning Source LLC
Chambersburg PA
CBHW060631290526
45793CB00001B/211